Understanding Self-Help/ Mutual Aid

Understanding Self-Help/ Mutual Aid

Experiential Learning in the Commons

THOMASINA JO BORKMAN

R RUTGERS UNIVERSITY PRESS
New Brunswick, New Jersey, and London

Library of Congress Cataloging-in-Publication Data

Borkman, Thomasina.
  Understanding self-help/mutual aid : experiential learning in the
commons / Thomasina Jo Borkman.
    p. cm.
  Includes bibliographical references and index.
  ISBN 0-8135-2629-9 (cloth : alk. paper). — ISBN 0-8135-2630-2
(pbk. : alk. paper)
  1. Self-help groups. I. Title.
HV547.B67 1999
361.4—dc21   98-50649
                                                                       CIP

British Cataloging-in-Publication data for this book is available from the British
Library

Manufactured in the United States of America

To my parents, Babe and Irene Stunz,
whose lives celebrated primary experience,
the entrepreneurial spirit, and an
ardent curiosity to understand their world

Contents

Preface

I FELL IN LOVE with a self-help group for people who stutter in 1970, when I was considering what research to embark on after my dissertation. The courage and determination that the people in the group showed, obviously frightened to speak yet speaking and stuttering anyway in a gathering they had convened, impressed me. My doctoral research on sociological correlates of social stress in relation to blood pressure levels in a representative sample had produced negative results, and I was disillusioned with the knotty complexities of conceptualizing, much less measuring, social stressors. The recognition that social support might mediate or buffer stress, and that the self-help group was an innovative, intriguing form of support—along with my fondness for the people who stuttered—convinced me to study them. This project expanded to include all the groups of people who stutter that I could locate in the United States as well as in New Zealand, Holland, and Sweden, thanks to a research grant from the National Institute of Mental Health.

In 1972 I joined a woman's consciousness-raising group and was nearly expelled because I initially communicated only with logico-scientific knowledge. (If sexism in the workplace was the topic, I brought in statistics about women's discrimination in pay for equal work or the equivalent.) This humbling experience taught me how to identify my own personal experience and talk about it in narrative form. As I participated in the group, I came to recognize that experiential learning and knowledge are essential parts of the foundation of self-help/mutual aid.

In the mid-1970s I reached a crossroads. Should I attempt to understand self-help/mutual aid on its own terms, regardless of where the journey took me across disciplines in search of appropriate concepts and methodologies, or should I commit to sociological formulations and work to develop them as theories and applied research? My entrepreneurial instincts—the interdisciplinary approach—won out.

My father was an entrepreneur who enthusiastically struggled with the challenges of creating new businesses but then lost interest and sold them when they were solidly established and running smoothly. Being my father's daughter, I have been trying to build an understanding of the fascinating social innovation of self-help/mutual aid. My research journey began in 1970 and has continued since then. I have received research grants to study groups and I have done research without special assistance. When appropriate I have attended meetings of various groups; when I encounter self-helpers I interview them; I read about them; I have informants who tell me about life in AA; I encourage my students to study them; I have friends and relatives in the recovery subculture. I have consulted for self-help groups, self-help resource centers, and government agencies. This book is the result of almost three decades of exploration and discovery.

One reviewer of a draft of this book said that I presented an "idealistic vision" of the self-help/mutual aid phenomena. This is true—I emphasize the best that self-help/mutual aid can be, and idealistic values underpin my work. Simultaneously, I try to be realistic and recognize that the best is often not realized in practice.

Not too long ago I was criticizing religion to a philosopher. He responded: what part of religion do you mean—are you talking about the best that religion can be, the worst that religion can be, or the middle? I am trying to show the best that self-help/mutual aid can be. Critics and self-help bashers emphasize the worst that it can be, but often without reference to facts or firsthand knowledge. Much of the academically based research on self-help/mutual aid can be classified as in the middle. Disciplinary conceptual frameworks, for example, chop human beings into cognitions, attitudes, and behaviors (and usually leave out the spiritual); studies assume that, like group therapy, the power of self-help/mutual aid lies in solely what goes on within the meetings, or that Yalom's eleven "therapeutic" factors found in psychotherapy groups provide the boundaries for looking at what works (L. Kurtz 1997). I think that the more rigorous the research that focuses on measurable factors within controlled conditions, the more mediocre the research will be in illuminating the self-help/mutual aid process. Self-help group participation is self-selected. Randomization is inappropriate. In contrast, I discuss the broader vision of the role of self-help/mutual aid in the qualitative and unmeasurable, in the innovative aspects of the "meaning perspectives" it creates, and in its contribution to democratic society. I try to show self-help/mutual aid's complexity rather than oversimplifying as many disciplinary-bound approaches do; I look for efficacious factors that Leonard Borman (1982) identifies as outside the therapists' control, not included in professional theories of what helps: instant identity, altruism or helping one another, networking and developing community, acquiring experientially based wisdom, and sharing information.

Underlying my analysis is a set of values and ideas that are critical of advancing professionalism, the overinstitutionalization of contemporary life (Ritzer's McDonaldization of society), and the withering of community. John McKnight (1995) is articulate in his critique of the dysfunctions of over-professionalizing life, turning society into a set of providers (the professionals) giving services to the dependent clients (the rest of us), labeling more and more people as defective or fallible with conditions that need treatment and service by professionals and the human service system. McKnight argues that three visions of society are implicit in the public discourse and in policymaking: the therapeutic vision, the advocacy vision, and the community vision. The therapeutic vision is the idea that an environment is composed of professionals and their services, developed in order to ensure the well-being of individuals; a professional is available to meet every need, and one has a "right to treatment" (1995, 169). The advocacy vision is an environment in which labeled people are protected by advocates and advocacy groups. It conceives of a defensive wall of helpers (legal advocates, support people, job developers, and housing locators) to protect an individual against an alien community; it seeks to ensure a person's right to be a functioning individual.

The community vision to which I subscribe is the associational one in which labeled and unlabeled people work together to emphasize one another's strengths and capacities. It sees the goal as "recommunalization" of exiled and labeled individuals. Community is understood as a basic context for enabling people to contribute their gifts. Strands of the community vision include: collective effort and shared responsibility, informal associations in which authentic relationships are possible and valuable transactions occur without money, advertising, or hype; stories, rather than studies or reports, convey the collective memories and wisdom; celebration, laughter, and singing. "The surest indication of the experience of community is the explicit common knowledge of tragedy, death, and suffering. . . . To be in community is to be an active part of associations and self-help groups. To be in community is to be a part of ritual, lamentation, and celebration of our fallibility" (McKnight 1995, 172). In my idealistic vision professionals provide specialized help to clients but are also human beings who acknowledge their limitations and learn from the experientially knowledgeable self-helpers about the phenomenology of living with an illness or predicament. The self-helpers are respected for their experiential knowledge and authority. They collaborate with professionals and agencies from a standpoint of dignity, responsibility, and equality, for only they can show the rest of society the innovative and positive ways of struggling through predicaments that they have learned.

Acknowledgments

As I sit in my study surrounded by books, articles, interview notes, study findings, critiques of chapters, and the like, I question how anyone can think she writes a book by herself. Thank you, the many self-helpers I listened to and whose groups I visited, for showing me your travails and triumphs, your caring and courage. My recovering friends who continually teach me about the intricacies of self-help/mutual help are, among others, Jeani N., Maggie B., Mary Ann S., Russ M., Lee C., Michael S., Marilyn M., John M., Sanci M., and John L. The names of self-helpers mentioned in the text are pseudonyms, as are the names of all the self-help groups for people who stutter.

I highly value the colleagues who have engaged me in challenging dialogues or provided thoughtful reviews of my recent work, including Asaf Zohar, Roger Lohmann, Lou Medvene, Carl Milofsky, Ken Schmitz, Mary Shivanandan, Lee Ann Kaskutas, Nancy Dixon, Brad Cox, John Stone, John Messer, Don Boileau, and Ken Perkins. And among the other colleagues who have also provided helpful reactions at different stages of this work I thank especially Francine Lavoie, Randi Fine, Vic Murray, Mark Jacobs, Mark Chesler, Mellen Kennedy, Keith Humphreys, Ernie Kurtz, Linda Kurtz, Victoria Rader, Nancy Hanrahan, Judy Wilson, Greg Meissen, David Horton Smith, Arthur Williamson, Ben Gidron, Barbara Stupp, and Mary Warren.

I am especially grateful to Aina Stunz for her special editorial assistance, organizing acumen, unwavering moral support, and enthusiasm for my ideas. I deeply appreciate my friend Richard Rashke's time and support in sharing his experiential wisdom about the process of writing a book—he was consistently on target. My family was also wonderful; my husband Placy graciously tolerated my messy work habits, resolved my computer problems, and used his emotional intelligence to keep me centered. At various stages I benefited from the computer skills and editorial help of Anna Jakubowski, Sarah Amsler, Doreen Valentine, Rebecca McGovern, Peter Slavin, and Rose Wellman. Most recently Elizabeth Gretz's gentle and smoothing hand has honed the entire manuscript; I have appreciated her perceptive comments and incisive improvements. And the usual disclaimer: I take responsibility for the blemishes and errors of this work in process.

Understanding Self-Help/ Mutual Aid

Chapter 1

What Is Self-Help/ Mutual Aid?

Wednesday evening, *seventeen people sit in a circle in a meeting room at a speech and hearing clinic in an eastern city. The president, Mick, a thirty-year-old who stutters and is a cofounder of the five-year-old group, leads the meeting. He announces that the topic tonight will be difficulties in talking on the telephone. Sam, age forty-five, who joined the group four years ago, says haltingly but confidently, "I ffound the tel-telephone the hardest-hardest thing, other than saying my own name! Mmy ststuttering gets worse on the phone. I-I take so long to get words out that people hang up. I-I have been humiliated, embarrassed, [made] angry by the way people treat me." John, a twenty-one-year-old who has been coming periodically for a year, sympathetically agrees. "I was glad to find that I wasn't alone—that you agonized [when] talking on the phone also." As they go around the circle, some choose not to speak. Others slowly tell personal anecdotes of their misery in making phone calls and the cruel reactions of some listeners who accuse them of being mentally retarded or high on drugs, or even hang up on them. Everyone listens sympathetically; no one interrupts or shows restlessness at even the slowest, most tortuous speech.*

"What can I do? Do I just keep avoiding the phone?" asks newcomer Sally, in a voice full of frustration. Sam empathetically tells of techniques he has heard about in the group over the past four years. Some worked for him, others did not. Mick agrees with Sam, then adds: "The two speech therapists I went to were not interested in helping me with my phone problem—I've gotten help here. In general, as I have become less afraid of stuttering and tried to hide it less, I am also not so disfluent on the phone." Jerry, a twenty-four-year-old who started coming occasionally three months ago, gets angry about the people who give unsolicited advice to "slow down

*or relax—you won't stutter if you aren't so nervous." Jerry continues, "I've been
stuttering since I was six years old—if it was as easy as relaxing or slowing down, I
would have stopped years ago." Ellen, a fifty-year-old who has come regularly for
three years, comments: "Well, those people don't stutter—how would you expect
them to know anything?"*

*The meeting ends with those present, in turn, saying their name, which they
agree can be one of the most difficult speaking tasks—"I am Sam," "I am Mick,"
and so on around the circle.*

THIS VIGNETTE, based on an actual self-help group meeting, illustrates a number of familiar aspects of self-help groups as they are commonly perceived. A
small number (usually less than twenty) of people with the same predicament,
disease, or disability sit in a circle, sharing personal stories of their suffering
and their attempts to cope with and resolve the problem. I refer to this intimate sharing of personal stories, which is informative, egalitarian, and supportive, as a "circle of sharing" or a "sharing circle." But this familiar portrait
of a self-help group meeting is incomplete: it leaves out the underlying and
surrounding context—the organizational, cultural, and institutional milieu in
which the group evolves.

All the participants stutter, they all have similar difficulties talking on
the telephone, and they openly express their intense feelings of rejection and
humiliation. Their talk is grounded in personal stories of actual encounters.
No one comments on survey statistics or polls; members do not discuss someone else's stuttering or a television show on stuttering. There is no quoting of
expert knowledge; to the contrary, Mick implicitly criticizes two speech therapists for disregarding his telephone troubles. Similarly, the commonsense advice of the "man on the street" is regarded as uninformed and unhelpful.
Participants such as Mick, Sam, and Ellen who have been in the group for
several years seem to be less bothered by their telephone troubles and speak
about how they have learned to deal with these problems, whereas Sally and
Jerry, relative newcomers, seem to have no answers and can only express anger and frustration. The old-timers have changed. The group has evolved a
framework or a liberating "meaning perspective" that views the problem of
stuttering in a way that is useful for problem solving and is life enhancing.

The social technology, that is, the structuring of social relations by which
people change, is the "sharing circle" and the narratives (or stories). In problem solving to combat the stigma and rejection from others, members have
evolved the social technology as a collective, which has resulted in a liberating meaning perspective that redefines their identify and destigmatizes them.

The group has become a "normal-smith" who assumes that people categorized by society as undesirably different are capable of rapid and wholesale change and of becoming essentially normal.[1]

The group in the vignette is a voluntary association with elected officers and members, a membership organization in which the people who stutter control and maintain the organization. Professionals or others who do not stutter are not allowed to be officers. No professional, government, or service agency operates or maintains the group. Yet it has been functioning for five years, which means that someone has been recruiting members, arranging meeting topics, negotiating a place to meet, and attending to the organizational needs that allow the group to function.

All of the questions raised by the vignette are addressed in this book.

> Who participates? Is pain a prerequisite for participation? How and why are participants willing to put aside their public façades and expose their vulnerabilities to one another? Is this just another form of the television and radio talk shows?
>
> What is the basis of knowledge and authority used in the group? What is the relationship to the public? To professional experts? What are the implications of the absence of a professional?
>
> To what extent did the group facilitate change in an individual's perspective? How do the participants help themselves and help one another? Are all attendees helped equally?
>
> What is the impact of hearing many similar stories from one's experiential peers? How is the collective knowledge of individuals and the group as a whole affected by the accumulated sharing of many people over a period of time?
>
> Who and with what authority or under what auspices has assembled this group? Who controls or maintains the group? How has the group developed and changed over time?

Two distinctions are key to appreciating and understanding self-help and mutual aid: primary lived experience and the voluntary commons. These two themes and their interrelationship are the focus of this book. The thesis can be succinctly summarized in three sentences:

> Situated within the voluntary and nonprofit organizations sector of American social-institutional life, self-help/mutual aid organizations function as consumer-controlled, adult-learning forums, peripheral to

professionally run institutions, where the "commons" space creates a distinctive agent of change through experiential-social learning.

The voluntary "commons" (Lohmann 1992) provides a space in which self-help/mutual aid can flourish (or languish) in a multiplicity of forms.

Individual self-helpers can evolve from self-pitying "victims," to self-determining survivors, or beyond to thrivors within these contexts; similarly, self-help organizations can also evolve through developmental phases.

A Tower of Babel? Naming Self-Help and Mutual Aid

We first need to understand the terms "self-help" and "mutual aid." Researchers and observers of self-help groups have struggled for years with the terms self-help, mutual aid, self-help group, mutual help group, support group, and related terms to express the same idea. Identical terms have been defined quite differently. In 1987 the Surgeon General's Workshop on Self-Help and Public Health, the major national-level policy event showcasing self-help and mutual aid, adopted the term "self-help group," even though it leaves out the idea of mutual aid because the term is so widely known by the public. But among the media, the public, and health and human service professionals and agencies, these terms are often used without clear definition.

"Self-help" will be distinguished from "mutual aid" in this book. Self-help will refer to an individual's taking action to help him- or herself, often drawing on latent internal resources and healing powers within the context of his or her lived experience with an issue or predicament. The process of struggle can result in individuals' taking responsibility for their behavior and becoming empowered, or not; some individuals retain their victim status and cannot rise above their misfortunes. This definition of self-help is similar to that used by Frank Riessman and David Carroll (1995). Self-help includes do-it-yourself techniques such as self-help books or tapes in an independent educational process.[2]

Self-help is contrasted with external interventions such as the physician who gives medication to ease pain or the teacher who lectures in a workshop on how to increase assertiveness. I will use "support group" to refer to professionally managed groups of people who have the same problem.

Mutual aid or mutual help refers to individuals joining together to assist one another either emotionally, socially, or materially. Mutual aid can be neighbors helping a family rebuild a home destroyed by fire or members of a self-help group listening to one another and providing emotional support. I will use "mutual aid" to refer to cases of reciprocal assistance whether or not self-help is present.

Joining these two concepts is the adage "you alone can do it but you cannot do it alone," often quoted in the literature on self-help and mutual aid. The expression frequently baffles critics of self-help groups. "You alone can do it" implies self-responsibility and independence, whereas "you cannot do it alone" implies mutual aid and dependence. Joining these two produces a special form of interdependence in which the individual accepts self-responsibility within a mutual aid context—individuals both maintaining independence while helping others, and receiving help from others. I will use the term "self-help group" to refer to this synergistic interdependence resulting from the combination of self-help and mutual aid as displayed by the opening vignette.

The widely respected American Self-Help Clearinghouse in New Jersey, directed by Edward Madara, prefers the term "mutual aid self-help" (MASH), but I find it awkward. Some researchers prefer the term "mutual help groups," but it leaves out self-help. The 1992 International Conference on Self-Help/ Mutual Aid in Ottawa chose the term "self-help/mutual aid" to encompass both aspects and to broaden the idea beyond groups and organizations to other forms such as buddy relationships or computer networks. I will use the term "self-help/mutual aid" as the most general term that encompasses both aspects in any and all organizational forms.

Self-help/mutual aid is primarily a grass-roots effort that emerges informally, often spontaneously, by and for the people who share a focal issue. Professionals may assist in the formation of groups, and some are initiated with the help of governments or health and human services agencies. Self-help/ mutual aid groups are richly diverse in their organizational formats, social technology, relations to professionals, and perspectives on their situation. Support groups controlled by professionals and operating under the auspices of hospitals or other human service agencies are far more structured than their consumer-controlled cousins; in fact, some self-help groups arise in reaction to support groups. For example, many breast cancer groups arose in reaction to the limited support available from the restrictive rules imposed by physicians who took control of the earlier self-help group Reach to Recovery.

In the last two decades, self-help groups, support groups, and associated self-help/mutual aid networks have expanded in frequency, type, and significance in the United States and other industrialized countries. According to a 1990 estimate, as many people attend experientialist-led self-help groups in a year in the United Sates as participate in professionally led psychotherapy (Jacobs and Goodman 1989). Nine percent of the United States population has attended an AA meeting (Room and Greenfield 1993). Even so, only 7.1

percent of the U.S. population or 2.4 percent of Canadians have attended self-help groups in one year (Kessler, Mickelson, and Zhao 1997; Gottlieb and Peters 1991).

Self-help groups appeal to those who join other voluntary associations and to those who are distressed about a problem or interested in actively resolving it within a group context. Twelve-step groups say that the program is not for people who need it but for people who want it. Some people have adequate support systems without a self-help group. In any case, self-help groups will always have a limited appeal, even though the reasons are not completely clear at this stage of research.[3]

Self-help resource centers or self-help clearinghouses have also evolved since the 1970s as an important interface between self-help groups and the public. All self-help resource centers in the United States act as information and referral agencies that maintain lists of self-help groups and provide the public or professionals with information on how to contact specific groups. Many resource centers also assist people in setting up new groups. Encouragement is a vital ingredient that resource centers can provide a new group, especially for rare diseases or conditions for which no model group exists, or inaccessible situations involving, for example, shut-ins, rural dwellers, or the physically disabled with transportation problems (Madara 1992).[4]

Self-help groups and self-help resource centers are a worldwide phenomenon, although more is known about them in industrialized democracies such as the United States, Canada, England, Germany, Israel, and Australia. In previously communist areas, such as Eastern Europe and the Soviet Union, self-help groups and self-help resource centers are being developed. Croatia, in the former Yugoslavia, has had groups for hypertension patients since 1976 (Barath 1990). Some African countries are developing support groups for people with AIDS and their families. One of the first International Conferences of Self-Help/Mutual Aid was held in Ottawa in September 1992. A special issue of the journal *Prevention in Human Services* and a book based on research papers presented at the conference were subsequently published (Lavoie, Borkman, and Gidron 1994).

Self-help groups of interest in the United States cover a multitude of life issues related to health and human services. There are groups formed around diseases (especially chronic illnesses), disabilities, other health issues, life transitions, relationship issues, and economic and social issues. Family members, friends, or significant others are the basis of many groups, such as Parents of Gay Children, Alliance for the Mentally Ill, Mothers of Twins Club, Parents of Murdered Children, Candlelighters, Al-Anon, and Tough Love. Groups are formed around lifestyles such as Parents without Partners, gay alliances, and

Gray Panthers or around transitions such as menopause, widowhood, breastfeeding, and terminal illness. Self-help groups that deal primarily with housing, economic, food, or other issues of material and structural aid have not been investigated as part of this study; however, many of the ideas presented pertain to them.

Also widely divergent is the "meaning perspective" or framework that develops in response to the same problem. Self-help groups can be oriented to all sides of an issue, a fact to which relatively little attention has been paid. An exception is Robert Emerick (1989, 1991), who has shown that groups for former mental patients or people in past psychotherapeutic treatment differ extensively along a continuum in their attitude toward the mental health establishment. At one extreme are strident rejecters of professional treatment, some of whom refer to themselves as "psychiatric survivors." At the other end of the continuum are those who endorse and cooperate with professional programs. To mention other examples, some self-help groups for overweight people accept the societal norms and values that favor slimness—these groups, such as TOPS (Take Off Pounds Sensibly), help members to lose weight. At the other extreme, groups such as Fat Is Beautiful reject the societal norms of slimness and advocate for changed values. Similarly, some groups for gays such as the National Gay and Lesbian Task Force help members accept their sexual orientation; other self-help groups such as Homosexuals Anonymous reject their sexual orientation and are trying to "live free from homosexuality" (White and Madara 1998, 274).

Self-help groups also vary in such organizational matters as goals, format, structures, phases of development, and longevity. These issues have not been well studied or understood. Alongside the well-known 12-step/anonymous groups are conventional voluntary associations, national networks of individuals linked by a newsletter and a yearly conference (such as Let's Face It, for individuals with a facial disfigurement), computer bulletin boards and online support groups, telephone peer relationships for people who are housebound or geographically scattered (such as people with rare diseases or the physically disabled), self-help agencies, and alliances of independent organizations. Self-help agencies that provide services, employ paid staff, have a significant budget, utilize self-help social technology instead of a professional approach, and rely on the experiential knowledge of self-helpers for organizational authority.[5]

The 12-step/anonymous programs are so distinctive in their combination of spirituality with self-help/mutual aid and in their organizational configuration that they need to be separated from other forms of self-help/mutual aid organized along conventional hierarchical lines.

The 12-step groups are well represented in the popular culture and are part of the community landscape across America.[6] The 12-step recovery programs evolved into a full-scale social movement by the end of the 1980s, according to Robin Room (1992). Examining the San Francisco Bay area, Room found networks of activities, organizations, magazines and newspapers, conventions, and recovery book stores devoted to the broader 12-step movement (as opposed to a focus on just one group, such as AA). Where AA and a few other groups like Al-Anon and Gamblers Anonymous stood alone in their practice of the 12 steps to recover from addiction or obsession with an addict, the field was now filled with hundreds of groups who embraced a wide set of issues as their focus of recovery. A publishing business in recovery-oriented books, tapes, and paraphernalia was thriving. Room maintains that the "shift in consciousness came in the wake of the growth of the Adult Children of Alcoholics (ACOA) movement. . . . ACOAs found themselves applying the 12 steps to general problems of living" (Room 1992, 718).

Self-help group researchers have categorized the groups in various ways, and each typology highlights some differences and obscures others. I propose a typology based on attributes of the self-help/mutual aid organization's "meaning perspective": (1) What does the meaning perspective say about the type and extensiveness of personal, identity, and lifestyle change (transformation) members should make in order to resolve their problem? And (2) what is the expected duration of participation in the group? Each attribute is dichotomized in terms of little or extensive transformation and short or long expected duration of membership; when cross-classified they result in a four-celled table.[7]

Little expected transformation refers to groups that help people cope with or adapt to stress, transition, or some affliction or condition that does not require an extensive personality, identity, or lifestyle change. A change of attitude, coping skills, and information may be needed along with social and emotional support during the process. Groups focused on transitions such as divorce, widowhood, or breastfeeding, relatively short-term caretaking, parents of gays, or parents of premature infants are examples. Extensive transformation is best exemplified by the 12-step/12-tradition groups for addictions. Other examples are groups for people who become blind or who become deaf, paraplegic, or suffer other permanent disabilities.

The degree of stigma (or social differentness and resulting awkwardness in social relations) societal groups attach to a condition, transition, or illness affects whether coping or transformation is needed. I argue that all self-help/mutual aid is formed in part in reaction against the stigma projected by others—friends, co-workers, strangers, professionals providing services, and so on—onto the shared problem that is the focus of the group. Mothers breastfeeding their babies may encounter some discomfort and awkward rela-

Table 1.1
Self-Help/Mutual Aid Typology

Expected scope of change	Expected duration of participation	
	SHORT	LONG
Small	Short-term coping 1	Long-term coping 2
Extensive	3 Short-term transformative	4 Long-term transformative

tions on the part of strangers or friends with whom they interact, but this mild stigma is unlikely to affect the mother's identity and overall lifestyle. But highly stigmatized conditions like blindness, alcoholism, or drug addiction affect the identity, lifestyle, opportunities, and life chances of the person so labeled. Highly stigmatized conditions create negative and self-hating identities; indeed, even certain mildly stigmatized conditions like stuttering affect some people who stutter very negatively—this is described in chapter 5.[8]

The second variable, expected duration of participation, is categorized as short or long. "Short" is defined as less than two years of expected participation by the average member; "long" is defined as more than two years to a lifetime. (I base this definition on my knowledge of various groups; empirical research can confirm the extent to which this definition fits.) Participants who become leaders of a group are likely to continue their involvement for a longer period of time than regular members. Length of participation is implied or explicitly suggested by the "meaning perspective." The 12-step/12-tradition groups for addictions often argue that the addictive tendency is lifelong and that personal and lifestyle change can be best accomplished by continuous participation in the group.

In table 1.1, cell 1 (short-term coping), at one extreme, applies to groups that regard their problems as short term. Their members require assistance in coping, not major changes on the part of the person. Examples are life transitions such as divorce, widowhood, breastfeeding, or some groups for significant others—parents of gays, for example, who are trying to accept their children's homosexuality. Cell 4 (long-term transformative) is at the other extreme—the problem is defined as chronic or long term, requiring extensive changes in a person's lifestyle, personality, and identity to adapt successfully to it. Many physical disabilities such as deafness, blindness, becoming paraplegic, addictions, and chronic diseases such as multiple sclerosis are included here. Cell 2 (long-term coping) groups, which believe that only coping and support are needed, but for a number of years, probably occur less frequently; Weight Watchers, the corporate-owned support group whose program is lifelong but whose chief objective is maintaining one's weight through use of the organization's food plan, fits this category. Many parent groups for those who have children with a chronic disease that persists a long time, but the problem requires coping more than extensive change on the parent's part (children with mental illness, gifted/learning disabled, muscular dystrophy, and so on), also fall in cell 2. Cell 3 (short-term transformative) groups, which believe that identity and lifestyle change are required to resolve the problem, but the process takes months, not years, are also less common. People who stutter, however, are an example. Usually if extensive personality, identity, and lifestyle change are seen as necessary to problem resolution, it is likely to take longer than two years.

This typology focuses on how the group defines the problem and solution, not on how an outsider defines them. The schema can alert the reader to the fact that there is extensive diversity in groups. Those dealing with the same problem—say, alcoholism—can define it very differently. AA is clearly in cell 4. A relatively new alcoholism self-help group, Rational Recovery, falls in cell 1; the expected length of participation is a year or less, and the problem is viewed as changing certain cognitions, not a change in identity, personality, or "way of life."

This typology implies major factors affecting the nature of activities in the group, the organizational issues and problems the group is likely to face, the kinds of commitment members will form to the organization, and the nature and extent of community formed around the group. It can also reveal the diversity among groups' "meaning perspective" for the same problem such as overweight or alcoholism.

Professional Power, Knowledge, and Authority

Public and professional recognition of self-help/mutual aid as a legitimate avenue of support increased significantly during the 1980s and early 1990s. Yet on the whole such groups are still misinterpreted and marginalized by society. Self-help has tenuous links with many parts of the mainstream health and human services systems. Alcoholics Anonymous is the major exception; its 12-step ideas have been incorporated into many alcohol and drug treatment programs, and many recovering alcoholics, with and without professional credentials, work in these programs.

Power and control are central issues in discussing mainstream health and social services systems and their linkages with self-help/mutual aid. For at least three decades, the social sciences have analyzed the impact of professionals as experts who have the power to control diagnosis, treatment, and services.[9] Physicians and other licensed health and social service professionals have the societally and legally mandated right to treat patients. These mandated relationships are essentially hierarchical, with the professional superordinate and the patient subordinate. The hierarchical differences is based partly on knowledge; the professional is the expert, which empowers him or her and disempowers the client—clients tend to become dependent on professionals. The relationship is basically contractual; the client or patient agrees to put him- or herself in the care of the professional for a designated problem in exchange for payment. The social distance between the professional and the client varies, but it is essentially a hierarchical one. The structure of this relationship is in stark contrast to the "sharing circle" of experiential peers in the self-help group. Accompanying the professional-client relationship are a series of other differences such as perspective and discourse.

Professionals increasingly operate in agencies, hospitals, and other bureaucratically based organizations that are themselves hierarchical and often owned or funded by for-profit corporations, health insurance companies, or governments. Their organizational work life is formal, procedure- and rule-based, and requires extensive paperwork and accountability. Self-help researchers contrast the professional relationship, with its bureaucratic organization, with the self-help ethos, which is, among other things, antibig, antibureaucratic, and collaborative, valuing democratic, shared decision making, informality, and experiential wisdom.

The predominance of professional institutions and the dominance of large-scale corporations in U.S. society at the turn of the twenty-first century are major features that affect policymaking, views of the "good society," competition for public monies, and the loyalties of citizens. John McKnight, in his book *Careless Community: Community and Its Counterfeits* (1995), summarizes some of these trends and suggests that public discourse is dominated by three visions: therapeutic, advocacy, and the community vision. The therapeutic vision is a world in which the environment is composed of the professionals and their services; they are oriented to the well-being of individuals who have the "right treatment." A professional is available to meet every need of the citizens. The advocacy vision is more adversarial, seeking to ensure a person's right to be a functioning individual. And the third vision of community is all-encompassing, enabling people to contribute their strengths and gifts to others without focusing on their fallibilities.

The postmodernists argue that American society has lost its grand narrative. The legitimizing force of the scientific and rational knowledge of the white male is crumbling, to be replaced by various multicultural groups—African-American, women, Hispanics, lesbians and gays—that have their own "voices" of truth, knowledge, and authority (Lyotard 1993). Nevertheless, the power of scientific knowledge as a source of truth is considerable in the medical profession. The helping professionals are regarded as the experts, especially in relation to the client.

On the broad canvas of American society at the close of the twentieth century, the professions reign in relation to their clients. The power and knowledge split between the professions and their clients is still huge, even while it has been diminishing since the 1960s. In the fields of health and human services, professionally based agencies, managed care insurance companies, and the government programs of Medicare and Medicaid, among others, are mammoth presences that command so many resources that they have an overwhelming influence in shaping the structure of opportunities within which individuals act. Although, the patient's bill of rights, ombudsmen and appeal mechanisms, the socialization of younger professionals to listen to their patients, more proactive health consumers, and other mechanisms have reduced the distance between the professional and the client, the power of professionals to define situations and diagnose and treat problems indicates that McKnight's "therapeutic vision" is entrenched.

Self-Help Bashing and Thoughtful Criticism

Along with the popularization and familiarization of self-help groups came a spate of "self-help bashing" (Riessman 1990a), which was frequently without substantiation. It perceived self-helpers as:

- Excessively emotional whiners like the complainers on television and radio talk shows
- Part of groups that exploit their members with high fees for workshops on their "inner child" and with books to buy from self-serving professionals or other proponents of their movement
- Part of groups wherein the "ignorant lead the ignorant"—lay people or newly diagnosed patients who know nothing about their chronic disease give one another advice
- Self-absorbed navel-gazers who do not address the social and economic problems of society that are causing their problem

- Victims who will not take responsibility for their own behavior
- Exhibitionists—emotional females as found on "women's" talk shows and magazines

In addition to the often vitriolic self-help bashing, some thoughtful and substantiated criticisms of self-help/mutual aid are found. Robert Wuthnow (1994), who extensively studied the small meaningful groups in which Americans participated in a large representative national sample, questioned the depth of "community" expressed by self-helpers. Wuthnow suggested that the available support was primarily emotional, not material, and that it was often tenuous and transitory. Further, he questioned the depth of the "spirituality" manifested by self-helpers in 12-step anonymous programs and other self-help groups with a spiritual basis; in comparison with the devoutly religious, he found the "spirituality" of self-helpers superficial.[10]

Some self-help bashing is based on misunderstandings of the nature of self-help/mutual aid. To begin with, the fact that self-help/mutual aid organizations are voluntary is critical. In voluntary forums, people choose the amount and kind of involvement they have with the group. Developed groups involve people with a common situation who can communicate information, wisdom, and hope regarding their predicament and find courage and strength from one another to resolve their shared issue in a constructive, life-enhancing way.

Critics characterize self-help groups as forums for whining victims or as social clubs without problem-solving agendas. These characterizations apply to some attendees, especially newcomers who sometimes behave as "victims," and to some fledgling or unsuccessful groups. These characterizations can also reveal a logical error made by the critic. How many critics talk to drop-outs or dissatisfied attendees of a group and then describe the collective on the basis of these unrepresentative participants, people who know the least about the group? Contrary to critics' claims, a major characteristic of effective self-help/mutual aid is that self-helpers learn to take responsibility for their actions as part of the healing and recovery process.

Another error is confusing for-profit self-help and voluntary self-help/mutual aid. John Bradshaw (1990, 1996), Melody Beattie (1989, 1990), and others have moved into the commercial sector and now trade on their recovery by selling workshops on the "inner child" or recovery books and tapes to make a living; the critics mistakenly lump them together with the voluntary giving that occurs in self-help groups.

Contrary to self-help bashing, in viable self-help groups, the committed participants face their shared problem and, in telling their stories, relive the pain, stigma, and other negative aspects of their situation in order to work through it with dignity. Those individuals who are willing to experience the anguish and negativity surrounding the shared problem receive support from the group, which aids them in resolving their problem or situation in a constructive, life-enhancing way. Within the group, at least, they "come out of the closet" about the focal problem. They explore their personal and social identities in light of their shared experience. Some examine what it means to be a human being.

Other people who attend the same self-help group occasionally, or who otherwise do not get intimately involved, are unlikely to receive much help from the process. The self-help/mutual aid process only works through involvement and participation. Unlike medications prescribed by a physician that work regardless of the attitude of the recipient, the more you are involved in sharing your story and helping others, the more help you will receive from the process.

The self-help group composed of voluntarily attending persons who consciously face a shared problem with the moral support of their peers stands in sharp contrast with many situations in which people with a similar problem are placed in physical proximity but with no sense of shared problem solving. For example, I have talked to professionals who see patients with similar problems lined up in their waiting rooms. I have interviewed people in such situations who were despairing and negative about their own problem; they were extremely upset to be near others like themselves. I recall the parents of a neurologically impaired child who was violent and difficult to manage. Seeing a number of other children behaving like their own child in the waiting room seemed to multiply, rather than alleviate, the parents' negativity and despair. In short, simply being in physical proximity with others who have shared the same experience is insufficient to produce the positive dynamics of a self-help group. The dynamics that operate in the medical waiting room are very different from those in self-help groups.

Viable self-help/mutual aid is goal-oriented and problem solving, but much of the "work" is emotional, interior, and applies to the invisible and mundane sphere of private life. The seeming paradox that the task-oriented problem solving revolves significantly around issues of feelings and meaning stems from a widespread assumption in our overly rationalized society that trivializes emotional work, regarding it as unimportant or not worthwhile. The demeaning of "caring" and emotional work is an attitude that feminists, among others, seek to counter.

The process by which both group members and the collective evolve a constructive worldview and "meaning perspective" is an important part of self-help/mutual aid. Self-help problem solving is a learning process in which individuals and collectives go through developmental phases based on primary lived experience.

Primary Experience: The Basis of Participation, Knowledge, Authority

Primary or first-hand experience with a predicament is the basis of (1) the individual's involvement as a person in self-help/mutual aid and the commonality of the people who meet together in the group, (2) the learning experience they undergo mutually and reciprocally to grapple with the common predicament, and (3) the individual's gain of experiential knowledge, self-determination, and self-authorization (trust in her knowledge of her experience and a voice about her predicament), (4) the group's evolution of a meaning perspective for the common predicament that has been "tested" against the personal experiences of participants and found to be helpful to the members, and (5) the group's evolution of an experiential authority base that legitimizes the experiential learning technology used by the group and validates the knowledge and wisdom gained from practicing it.

Individuals participate as whole persons, as a unity: a physical body with mental capacities, emotions and feelings, a social identity, and spirit (which encompasses meaning and hope). In contrast with segmental roles (for example, being the patient with their physician or the client with professional staff), in self-help/mutual aid an individual's personality is known to others by the display of her feelings, her innermost and private shame, her anger and guilt. Public façades are dropped, often within a context of anonymity where revelations are kept confidential by others. The vulnerability, sharing, and intimate exposure takes place within a situation of reciprocal and mutual exchange. This safe situation is in sharp contrast to the public exhibitionism of television talk shows. In chapter 2, I describe the participant as a unified person, borrowing from philosophy some concepts of the person and considering issues of human agency to examine how individual self-helpers and self-help groups can evolve from victims into self-determining and self-authorizing entities.

A central distinguishing feature of the self-help group is the reliance on information and wisdom gained from working through one's personal experience of the problem in a network of experientially similar peers. This experientially grounded knowledge becomes a major basis of authority in the group.

Experiential knowledge is truth based on personal experience with a phenomenon rather than information gained by hearsay, folk or lay knowledge, professional knowledge, or the pronouncements of a charismatic leader. Not all people who undergo an experience become knowledgeable about it (Borkman 1976). They do not develop a coherent sense of the experience, cannot use what they learned from it, and cannot articulate what they know because of having undergone the experience.

A reflective process is necessary to convert "raw experience"—which is often a jumble of inchoate images, thoughts, impressions, and feelings—into meaningful knowledge, which implies some form, coherence, and meaning. The reflective process can be experienced by oneself or with others. A key point about self-help groups is that the reflective process occurs with others who have shared the same experience and thus have specialized information about it and a personal stake in its interpretation. This communal learning can produce "collective experiential knowledge," which is qualitatively different from one person's idiosyncratic interpretation of his experience. Moreover, the voluntary context of peers' problem solving for the benefit of the participants provides significantly different dynamics than those created by political action advocacy or the promotion of one's financial position or career.

The social technology of helping members is based on experiential-social learning; the group provides a setting in which people can learn from their own and others' experiences. Members are adults who are willingly choosing to do something about a problem that they find, in the case of stuttering, to be persistent, upsetting, stigmatizing, and that interferes with their functioning. Stigmatizing conditions spoil or damage the identity of the labeled persons.

Self-help group participation is often accompanied by the use of professional services who help with technical aspects of the problem. But the group encompasses the whole person in her spiritual, emotional, physical and mental aspects. In the group described in the vignette, for example, a speech therapist, a professor in the university housing the speech and hearing clinic, had a role in initiating the group and had obtained the right for members to hold their meetings in the clinic without charge; his involvement had decreased over time as he saw that the group had become self-sustaining. Self-helpers often become sophisticated and discerning patients or service recipients—they know what professionals have to offer and what they can expect from them. They learn the limits of professional knowledge.

The "meaning perspective" or framework of the group about the shared predicament is key to linking the potential participant with the group. The potential participant, an adult, has a worldview or set of beliefs, values, and ideas about his predicament and life. Is the group's viewpoint about the predicament acceptable or not to the potential participant? If the discrepancy in viewpoints is too extensive, the person is unlikely to participate in the group.

Well-developed self-help groups like Alcoholics Anonymous or Recovery, Inc., have a coherent meaning perspective that provides guideposts about the nature of the common predicament, its possible resolution, and how to achieve it. Successful self-help/mutual aid organizations evolve life-enhancing meaning perspectives that encompass all aspects of the person who is participating. The voluntary commons setting facilitates this evolution, because in it there are no competing demands either from professionals to limit these meaning perspectives to their often-technical point of view or from corporations who need to make a profit from these activities.

The Voluntary Commons: Social Container of Self-Help/Mutual Aid

The social-institutional context in which self-helpers meet, learn, and evolve is known as the "third sector," or the voluntary action and nonprofit sector. The voluntary action or third sector also reflects a multidisciplinary field of research and practice. Government or the state constitute the first sector, for-profit business and the marketplace of capitalism constitute the second sector, voluntary associations of all kinds as well as nonprofit organizations constitute the third sector, and households and families constitute the fourth sector. Different values, laws, sanctioning systems, and institutional patterns obtain in the various sectors.

The group for people who stutter described in the opening vignette is an instance of a commons. The commons is a space in the third sector in which participants share a common purpose, hold something in common, and participation is mutual, free, and uncoerced, based in fairness (Lohmann 1992). The commons encompasses the informally organized self-help group in someone's living room, a self-help conference, or a one-time activity as well as more formally organized groups that are legally incorporated and have budgets.

The social science literature on self-help/mutual aid has taken a disproportionately therapeutic and individualistic perspective, focusing on such questions as how individuals are benefited by their participation in a group. Issues of group dynamics within self-help/mutual aid have been examined either from the perspective of group therapy controlled by a professional or as alternative human services within which the self-help groups' similarities and differences with professional services were examined.

The voluntary action perspective adds an expanded viewpoint and a rich literature on which to draw. Framing self-help/mutual aid phenomena as operating in the voluntary or third sector will reveal more about how they operate as organizations, and how they not only help their members but benefit society than viewing them simply as alternative forms of group therapy or human services. Many new and additional organizational questions regarding how they emerge, develop, and flourish or languish can be raised from this third sector perspective. Even the question of how individuals benefit can be expanded to include the issue of how contributing to the maintenance of the organization enhances or detracts from the benefits received.

To demonstrate the insights to be gained from adopting a voluntary action perspective of self-help/mutual aid organizations we can ask the following questions. On what basis are people involved in the group? What are the types and patterns of participation? What are the participants' relationships to one another? In voluntary associations, participants choose when and how often to attend and what level of involvement to have. Relationships are based on "moral" rather than "utilitarian" or "coercive" grounds; individuals participate because they agree with the values and goals of the group, what it stands for and is trying to achieve for its members. Little money is involved in the self-help/mutual aid organization, in contrast with the for-profit business sector, where utilitarian material gain and career advantage are major currencies. The mutual aid—listening, support, and emotional help—is a gift voluntarily offered, rather than an exchange relationship to enhance one's career prospects. People contribute primarily their time, attention, and personality (Perrow 1970) as they wish.

The voluntary commons provides multiple opportunities for a variety of types of participation and involvement, from a one-time contact to the other end of the continuum: a new way of life in an experientially based community. Unlike professionally controlled support groups that tend to be closed (no new participant is allowed after a cutoff date) and of a fixed duration (such as eight or twelve sessions), self-help/mutual aid is usually open, with newcomers entering a group in which members participate with varying frequency and for different lengths of time.

From a voluntary action perspective, self-help/mutual aid is a new form of volunteering in which people not only help others (as would a conventional volunteer) but receive help in the process (the equivalent of a consumer). Frank Riessman (1965), in a well-known article, described the "helper therapy" principle as a powerful agent of change in self-help groups; the principle is that the helper is receiving more aid in the process of assisting another than the recipient. More recently, Alvin Toffler (1980) captured the essence of the new volunteerism with the concept of the prosumer. The term "prosumer" indicates that the self-helper is both a "provider" of services to others in the group and a "consumer" of services from others. How are these new volunteers similar to and different from conventional volunteers? Many questions asked about conventional volunteers have not been asked of these new volunteers.

I will show that using the voluntary commons perspective illuminates the way in which it is a social space for innovation in form, structure, and type that produces a variety of new organizational forms (that is, learning organizations and self-help agencies). For example, self-help agencies provide services in exchange for fees but rely primarily on the experiential knowledge of self-helpers rather than on the typical rational-legal authority of the bureaucracy or the professional authority of the professional.

In what ways, if any, does participation in self-help/mutual aid affect self-helpers functioning in civil society? Do self-helpers' organizational experience provide skills and capacities for more effective participation in democratic institutions? What do these groups contribute to social capital, to social change or resistance to it, and to stability or renewal in society? These questions have rarely been raised.

Locating self-help groups within the social-institutional context of the third sector also raises issues of how self-help and mutual aid articulates with and interfaces with government policy and programs, professionally based services, or proprietary interests. What are the relationships and roles of government, professional agencies, and for-profit firms in enhancing or detracting from self-help groups and organizations? A critical issue: Do the institutionalized, and often rich and powerful, mainstream players help or detract from self-help/mutual aid by providing resources? Under what conditions do they try to control and subvert or facilitate the self-help/mutual aid process?

Perspectives: Professional, Experientialist, and Layperson

People living with a problem have the capacity to develop experiential knowledge and wisdom about their situation by participating in self-help/mutual aid. This experiential perspective is different from that of the involved professional or lay bystander, partly because of the different relationship each has to the problem.

Three perspectives are important to distinguish: (1) the professional is trained to diagnose and treat the problem but also has financial and career interests in it; (2) the experientialist is the person living through the problem firsthand; and (3) the layperson is a bystander who has secondhand information about it and has no interest or stake in the problem. Each perspective generates its own form and body of knowledge and understandings.[11]

Jerome Bruner has proposed two modes of cognitive functioning or thought: the logico-scientific and the narrative or story. Each has a distinctive way of ordering experience and of constructing reality; they are irreducible to each other. Each has its own operating principles, criteria of well-formedness, and procedures for verification. Both can be used to convince someone but of different things: the logico-scientific argument convinces one of its truth; narrative is the ideal form to convey meaning. The logico-scientific mode, which has been developed over hundreds of years, has its own aids: logic, mathematics, science. At a macro level it deals with general causes, and looks for the universal. The logico-scientific mode uses agreed upon procedures to empirically test hypotheses. An imaginative application of this mode of thought leads to good theories, tight analysis, logical proof, sound argument, and empirical discoveries based on sound methods (Bruner 1986, 11–13).

In contrast, the imaginative application of the narrative mode leads to good stories, gripping dramas, believable though not necessarily true historical accounts. The narrative mode is built on concern for the human condition; it deals in human intention, human action, and life's vicissitudes. Bruner argues that the narrative mode must construct two landscapes: one of action and one of consciousness. The constituents of action involve agent, intention or goal, situation, instrument and "something corresponding to a 'story grammar'" (Bruner 1986, 14). The language of consciousness pertains to what those involved in the action think, know, or feel or do not think, know, or feel. A gulf between the self-helper experientialist and the professional is grounded in the different modes of thought each primarily relies upon to do work. Biomedical discourse is based on the logico-scientific method whereas self-helpers create and transmit meaning through stories.

Biomedical discourse is one form of application of the logico-scientific mode that pertains to the general scientific laws, the maxims (for example, "first, do no harm"), statistical regularities, and the biomedical discourse by which cases are entered in patient's files or discussed in medical rounds. Cheryl Mattingly (1991) calls this discourse "chart talk" that is centered around the diagnosis, not the person. The presentation of a case follows its own rules that exclude much of the particularity of the patient. The focus is on issues surrounding the diagnosis and associated treatments for it. The case becomes a number with a specific diagnosis and treatments.

In contrast, analysts who study narratives or stories emphasize that human experience is rendered meaningful through the narrative or storytelling mode.[12] Self-help groups communicate through stories to convey experience, transform identity, and re-create an alternative social world as well as to create the group's liberating meaning perspective. The narrative mode centers on an individual person in his or her concrete and unique circumstances and particularity. Mattingly shows that storytelling and story analysis can facilitate a kind of reflection that considers the ordinarily tacit assumptions and ideas that guide practice; this reflective work is part of the sharing circle (Mattingly 1991, 236).

The professional is defined here as a college-credentialed and licensed occupational specialist who is knowledgeable about the diagnosis and treatment of the specific problem in question.[13] If one's training does not include knowledge about breast cancer, then the individual is not a professional vis-à-vis breast cancer. Professionals are trained to assess and identify a problem, and select and apply treatments or other solutions. Professional ideologies shape their views of a situation, and their training provides a suggested strategy to resolve the problem as they define it. Their training also prepares them to limit their emotional involvement; "detached concern" is the term that sociologists use. Despite the rhetoric that professionals are oriented toward serving and protecting their clients, professionals have occupational and personal interests, such as making money, winning prestige, and enhancing their careers.

The person experiencing the problem firsthand has a different set of interests in the way the problem is defined and the strategies to resolve it. He or she is personally experiencing it physically, mentally, emotionally, spiritually, with his or her social networks and identity and material interests involved. The experientialists suffer with the effects of the problem per se (whether it is the pain and disability from a rare chronic disease, the grief and disruption attending a spouse's death, or the daily effort of caring for one's granddaughter), and they undergo the effects of stigma, that is, not being regarded by others as a fully normal competent adult but treated to a greater or lesser extent as undesirably different (Goffman 1963). With highly stigmatized conditions, prejudice and discrimination can substantially reduce an individual's life opportunities. The experientialists react in different ways to the situation. Those who do not see the issue as problematic, or who are in denial of their problem, or who are not interested in problem solving about it are unlikely to be interested in self-help groups. They may turn over the responsibility for resolving their situation to the professionals and agencies treating them. But those experientialists who are concerned about problem solving or who are not in denial about their situation are more likely to choose self-help groups. The self-helper has the right to be intensely involved in decision making about his problem, and many self-help groups assist him in taking responsibility for actively participating in problem resolution. The passion and zeal of the self-helper can be misinterpreted; she is responding vigorously to threats to her self-interest, something professionals do as providers but in a more covert and emotionally controlled manner.

The experientialist, a person living firsthand with a problem, is usually thought of as the woman with breast cancer, the child with cerebral palsy, or the husband facing a divorce. But another category of person is living with the problem because of his or her close relationship to the person with the focal problem. The spouse, lover, parent, sibling, other relative, or close friend can be as subjectively involved as the person directly suffering the problem; in fact, these individuals' "problem" is partly their loved one who has the illness or predicament. They have interests and stakes in the way the problem is defined and resolved. Many self-help groups have been started for and by them: Al-Anon, for family members and friends of someone with an alcohol problem, the National Alliance for the Mentally Ill, Mothers of Twins Clubs, and so forth. These groups develop experiential perspectives and knowledge that overlap with but are also somewhat different from the person with the problem or situation. Frequently the person with the problem and their significant others are welcomed into the same self-help group; for example, medical self-help groups, such as ostomy groups or stroke groups, meet with both the sufferer and the spouse.

The third perspective is that of the layperson who has no professional training or firsthand experience with the problem. The layperson is the neighbor or member of the general public who is a bystander to the situation. Traditionally, the literature on self-help groups lumped together the lay bystander with the experientialist with the problem (or his/her significant other). The reference point was the professional, who was seen as significantly different from the undifferentiated others—clients and laypeople. But the bystander has no immediate stake in the problem nor any emotional or occupational interest in it. Lay bystanders rely on folk knowledge, which is a mixture of hearsay, information received secondhand from professionals, the media, or experientialists (who know the problem firsthand), or "recipe knowledge," that is, ideas passed down from one generation to another (Berger and Luckmann 1967).

Some people have multiple perspectives as both professional and self-experienced, such as the nurse with breast cancer or the psychotherapist who becomes widowed. We know little about how the two forms of knowledge intersect or complement one another.

Much experiential knowledge pertains to a different sphere than that of technical and specialized professional knowledge. The experiential perspective deals more with everyday life, the private lateral sphere of relationships and life maintenance, as Peggy McIntosh (1983) characterizes it, or with the existential and philosophical spheres involved in life's meaning and personal identity. The differences between the experiential and professional perspective are great. The experientialist reacts as a total human being to the problem or situation at hand; the professional has limited specialized interest in and knowledge of the problem. The experientialist is rooted in his or her subjectivity and is more explicitly emotional than the professional, who has been trained to control and manage emotional reactions. An important part of the experientialist perspective is to deal with one's feelings and emotions. Self-helpers do not merely think they know about how to deal with their problem. Gaining from collective sharing, hammering out a perspective, testing it against their embodied experience, they come to know they know.

Chapter 2
Experiential Learning in a Voluntary Commons

I was in the most extreme emotional pain in my life.
Some suggested I go to this group on Sunday night. I was
not exploring alternatives, investigating purposes,
reading mission statements. The group was a rope
thrown to a floundering swimmer—I grabbed it. At the
first meeting people, suffering pain like I was, were
there. I was not alone. That realization that there were
people with faces and names floundering like me was
enough.

— Wally, mid-forties, facing divorce

ACCOMPANYING Wally's emotional pain were physical upset, sadness, and despair, and a challenge to his meaning system as a practicing Catholic. His entire way of life was disrupted—his self-identity as a stable married father, his financial and housing situation, and his social relationships with friends and family.

The kind of help he could receive from various help-givers available in his community was fragmentary, segmented. His physician would be willing to listen to stories of insomnia and upset stomach but would have no interest in his housing problems; his attorney would probably become impatient hearing about his insomnia; his real estate agent would be indifferent to his spiritual anguish; his priest would have little practical or technical support to offer. His family, friends, and co-workers would offer general emotional support but with little in-depth understanding and probably little technical support. This man went to a self-help group in anguish, finding others who were sharing similar stories with the "language of the heart." He felt understood by them and, therefore, experienced a kinship with them. He received specific emotional support from others who were undergoing similar experiences; moreover, he received information about how to deal with the professionals, spiritual help in feeling estranged from Catholicism, and concrete suggestions for handling the myriad details of everyday living his altered roles thrust upon him (for example, how much water to put on the kitchen floor when washing it or how to cut up a whole chicken). Individuals thus participate in self-help/mutual aid organizations as whole persons, as unified wholes, rather than in segmental roles conforming to professionals' division of reality.

A person has a physical body, mind, emotions and feelings, and spirit or soul. He or she is an individual who searches for meaning and has free will to solve problems, make choices, and engage in action. Further, a person as a social being has a worldview, history, social identity, life plan, and network of relationships. The whole is greater than and different from the sum of its parts. This chapter will discuss the philosophical, sociological, and psychological bases of this theme. It will also examine how the lived experience—the basis of the predicament—is used as learning and "education" in self-help/mutual aid and why the voluntary sector model allows a fuller and more complete understanding of these organizations.

The Self-Helper: A Whole Person

Contemporary life and institutions have developed extreme specialization and an extensive division of labor. As patients, we approach specialists who focus on one organ system (the cardiologist or the endocrinologist, say) or one facet of our selves (the psychotherapist or the personal trainer). As customers, workers, or citizens we play other segmental roles. Philosophy has traditionally divided the human being in dualistic terms: Descartes is known for the mind/body dualism that modern science has continued. Psychology, following Descartes and others, often assumes that the physical senses are mediated by the brain, and that therefore mental activity is the real seat of our sensing of the world (Reed 1996b). Cognition or mental activity is separated from emotions or feelings. Until recently, much sociological theory left out the body; even the sociology of health and illness defined the subject matter in terms of the perspectives of various role players: what the physician thinks and does, what the patient perceives and does. For the social and physical sciences, the spirit or soul has been relegated to the province of religion, which, in a secularized society, is a form of invisibility.[1]

In contrast with the specialization and segmentalism inherent in contemporary society, many self-helpers find self-help/mutual aid organizations to be an arena where they are received as subjects, not objects, and where all facets of their selves can be revealed; where they are, indeed, whole persons.

THE PHILOSOPHICAL CONCEPT OF PERSON

I will be drawing on the concept of the human person developed by Kenneth Schmitz. In "Geography of the Human Person" (1986), Schmitz conceives of the human person as unique, a spiritual being with dignity and a capacity for intimacy as well as possessing a will to make choices and to take action.[2] "It is upon the uniqueness of each person and the diversity of all that human dignity rests" (Schmitz 1986, 27). The sense of a person as possessed of dignity and uniqueness, the capacity for intimacy and relationships of depth, and the capacity to participate with others in relationships involving appreciation and other intangible values, not just physical presence, is vital to understanding the process of self-help/mutual aid.

Schmitz traces the meanings of "person" historically and culturally to several sources and regions. One sense of the person is found in the comment that an authority figure treats us "as a person." "By that, we mean that he or she respects us and accords us a particular dignity and value; he or she shows interest in us, not out of curiosity, but intrinsically 'for ourselves'" (Schmitz 1986, 27). Our fundamental idea of a human being includes the capacity for feelings of tenderness and compassion, feelings closely associated with what we call "personal." The dignity of a person lies in being a spiritual being. Therefore, a person must always be treated primarily as an end in herself, not as a means or an instrument to satisfy another's wishes. A human being can only truly have "personal" relations with another human being, that is, one that recognizes this aspect of freely giving herself and accepting another in friendship or love (Schmitz 1986, 35).

Schmitz argues that "intimacy is the ontological locus out of which all other personal values take their rise, for this unique presence is the root of personal and therefore of distinctively human dignity" (1986, 45). Intimacy cannot develop in a dominating-submissive relationship but requires more equal relations in an atmosphere of trust.

> Intimacy arises within the circle of giving and receiving, and so it is
> not without a certain risk, the risk of self-rejection that is inseparable
> from the generosity of the gift of self. Intimacy is possible only
> through self-disclosure. Our intimate knowledge of a person is
> grounded in this act of mutual self-disclosure. . . . Intimacy is rooted
> rather in the unique *being present* of a person; and the principal mark
> of intimacy is *attentiveness to the presence of another.* (Schmitz 1986, 41)

Since the basis of self-help/mutual aid is undergoing similar primary experiences, and primary firsthand experience is by definition an integrated whole, the conception of personhood in this book needs to encompass all aspects of individuals as occurs in self-help groups. Rather than the typical differentiation among body, emotions, thoughts, and soul made in most Western philosophy, a whole person is defined as an integrated whole: a biological physical being with a body; an emotional being with feelings that are more or less integrated with and shape one's thoughts; an intellectual being with the functions of memory and reason; a spiritual being who uses his or her will to choose and to take actions or engage in behaviors.

The whole person is fundamentally a social being who exists in and because of her relations with other persons and the larger social world; we see this formulation of individuals as essentially social beings in the work of the pragmatist philosopher John Dewey; the social interactionist George Herbert Mead, a colleague of Dewey's at the University of Chicago; William James, the psychologist whose work Dewey respected and used; and of course most sociologists.[3] As a social being, a person is located in social and cultural space and time; for example, Maria Hernandez, a fictional person, is a Hispanic female born in Los Angeles, California, July 14, 1955, with a specific family background and current and past social relationships. From the social viewpoint one can characterize an adult person as having a worldview, a life plan, a personal and social identity, and a network of relationships, among other things. Race, social class, and gender are critical aspects of our social identity that affect our life chances and opportunities in the United States; historically white middle-class (or property-owning) males have been the generic "man" in Western thought and have disproportionately occupied and controlled elite positions in major social institutions. People of color, the lower class, and women have been the "Others," with restricted life chances and opportunities, whose voices and perspectives have been submerged or invisible (Collins 1993).

Social scientists conventionally deal with the mental-subjective, the emotional-feeling, and the social spheres. Fewer social scientists are used to dealing with the physical-bodily aspects of a person, since they are excluded as unimportant in many theoretical schemas. But in considering a human being as a whole person in the health and social arena, the fact that a person *is* a body, that is, in part she *is* her body (McCowan 1978) and in some contexts one *has* a body (Lupton 1994), is relevant. For example, he *is* a living body weighing 180 pounds with a set of teeth, a pancreas, a liver, and a functioning brain stem. He *has* a body in that he consciously watches his weight, brushes his teeth, periodically undergoes blood tests to determine whether his pancreas is producing insulin, and avoids excessive alcohol consumption out of concern for his liver. The biological physical being with a body has a genetic heritage, physiological idiosyncrasies and habits, capabilities or disabilities, and needs (such as wears glasses, limps in one leg, and can swim ten lengths of an Olympic-size pool). In the 1990s some theorists have been undertaking interdisciplinary work that connects the body, mind, and emotions or body, mind, and soul.[4]

SPIRITUAL ASPECTS OF THE PERSON

Since the spiritual aspect of a whole person is the least likely facet to be considered by conventional social science, I will deal with it in more detail. Mainstream social science disciplines, especially positivistic-based schemas, often define "person" by excluding the spirit or soul. The "spiritual" is so critical to understanding self-help/mutual aid, however, that it must be included in spite of the biases of some readers.

The usual meanings of spirit or spiritual found in self-help mutual aid seem to be associated with (1) the life principle, (2) orientation to spiritual ideas, (3) religion, and (4) disposition. These meanings of the words "spirit" and "spiritual" are based on the way they are used in 12-step programs and other self-help groups and related social science literature. I also contrast spirituality with therapy.

SPIRIT AS LIFE PRINCIPLE. Ernest Kurtz and Katherine Ketcham in *The Spirituality of Imperfection* (1992) say that human beings are inherently spiritual just as they have physical bodies. An analogy Kurtz and Ketcham use clarifies the meaning: a modern spiritual writer describes the spiritual as analogous with health. We all have health—some have good health, others, poor health. Health is something we cannot avoid having. Spirituality is the same in that all human beings are spiritual beings (Kurtz and Ketcham 1992).

ORIENTATION TO THE SPIRIT. The orientation toward or the *object* of these spiritual faculties is also a part of spirituality. To know and to love the inanimate world is different from knowing and loving another human being and/or God. The alcoholic "knows and loves" the bottle so that his spiritual faculties are skewed (Shivanandan 1994). Whether one's spirituality is negative, which leads to isolation and self-destruction, or positive, that is, more life giving, can vary (Kurtz and Ketcham 1992, 17). Thus we need to distinguish what is the focus and orientation of one's spiritual faculties (Shivanandan 1994).

A person's current orientation toward the spiritual versus the material world is often expressed in 12-step meetings. For example, someone might say, "I haven't been very spiritual lately," by which he might mean that he has attended to the everyday physical material world but neglected meditation and prayer and has not been grateful for intangible gifts such as friendship. Rachel

Naomi Remen, in her article "On Defining Spirit" (1993), expresses the orientation as the sense that human beings have the need to be spiritual, that is, as a potential, but not all human beings satisfy their need through their thoughts or action.[5] Remen seems to be referring to positive spirituality rather than spirituality as an essence that can be positive or negative, as Kurtz and Ketcham treat it. Remen says that it is difficult to define the "spiritual" directly and easier to say what it is not. She indicates that the spiritual is often confused with the moral, but morality is concerned with issues of right and wrong behavior and often used in making judgments that separate one individual or group from another. In contrast, the spiritual is profoundly nonjudgmental and inclusive. The spiritual is not within time but is unchanging. Moreover, the spirit should not be confused with the ethical, which "defines the right way to relate to other people, to carry out business and to behave in general. If the moral is not the spiritual, then the ethical isn't either." Third, the spirit is often regarded as part of the psyche, which is a way of perceiving:

> How I use what I see or hear, what it means to me, is what makes it a matter of spirit or not. I can use the psyche as I can use my other senses—to impress others, to accumulate personal power, to dominate or manipulate—in short to assert my separateness and my personal power. The spiritual however is not separative. A deep sense of the spiritual leads one to trust not one's lonely power but the great flow or pattern manifested in all life, including our own. We become not manipulator but witness. (Remen 1993, 41)

We participate in the moral because we are bodily beings and need to relate in concrete ways to the spiritual and to other human beings; although the moral cannot be separated from the spiritual, the moral rules are a way of manifesting spiritual principles (Shivanandan 1998).

SPIRITUALITY IS NOT RELIGION. Self-help groups usually separate their "spirituality" from religion, as do Kurtz and Ketcham, Remen, and others. Some explicitly Christian self-help groups may not separate religion and spirituality in the same way.

Kurtz and Ketcham, for example, following the 12-step philosophy, say the spiritual is not the same as the religious—"to the religious, spiritual seems soft, fluid, without boundaries. . . . To the spiritual who are not religious, religion seems full of doctrine, beliefs, boundaries, and us against them attitudes" (1992, 24–26). Remen also says the spiritual is not the religious. A religion is a dogma, a set of beliefs about the spiritual and a set of practices that arise out of those beliefs. There are many religions, and they tend to be mutually exclusive. That is, every religion tends to think that it has exclusive claim on the spiritual—that it is the one true way. Yet the spiritual is inclusive. It is the deepest sense of belonging and participation. We all participate in the spiritual at all times, whether we know it or not.

Remen expresses the connection between the spiritual and the religious: "The spiritual is that realm of human experience which religion attempts to connect us to through dogma and practice. Sometimes it succeeds and sometimes it fails. Religion is a bridge to the spiritual—but the spiritual lies beyond religion. Unfortunately in seeking the spiritual we may become attached to the bridge rather than crossing over it" (Remen 1993, 41). Clinging to the bridge, the religious person becomes more attached to the rules rather than to the purpose of the rules, which is spiritual (Shivanandan 1998).

DISPOSITION. There is a third sense of spirit that is central to self-help groups that has to do with one's disposition (this meaning is also implicit in Kurtz and Ketcham's definition of the spiritual). Many people come to mutual help groups discouraged, "depressed" to varying degrees about their situation, full of self-pity, hopeless, even suicidal. This negativity of spirit (disposition) is common, especially among newcomers. It is also expressed as unwillingness or lack of willingness to change or to take actions that will improve one's outlook or situation.

The 12-step programs emphasize that "we share our experience, strength, and hope." How that sharing is accomplished relates partly to the way in which conversation is structured in the meetings. Much of the group dynamics and interpersonal relationships in self-help groups pertain to caring about others as human persons in a nonjudgmental atmosphere. Some participants and observers believe that the crucial healing ingredients are listening with respect, compassion, and positive regard for the individual as a unique person of dignity in a nonjudgmental setting. Respect, listening, and caring are a way of sharing "strength and hope" that can reduce the "negativity of spirit" if the person is receptive to it.

SPIRITUALITY IS NOT THERAPY. Kurtz and Ketcham (1992) contrast the emphasis of a spiritual approach with that of a therapeutic one. The two approaches may be confused with each other because they both deal with healing and "making whole." However, they are based on different assumptions, metaphors, and discourses. The spiritual approach predominates in the 12-step/12-tradition groups although that is not often the case with other self-help/mutual aid organizations, especially those dealing with medical conditions or those devoted to social advocacy.

Therapy, which is integral to the therapeutic vision of society, has become scientific, demands proof, and focuses on technique and measurement. Therapy offers explanations and looks to etiology or causes "to push forces that compel, as the psychological language of 'drives' and the sociological focus on 'the shaping environment' attest" (Kurtz and Ketcham 1992, 27). Therapy relies on the medical metaphor, using the discourse of illness—sick, dysfunctional, unhealthy. Therapy's goal is happiness in the contemporary sense of feeling good.

Spirituality in contrast offers forgiveness, not explanations. Instead of "push forces" that imply a diminished sense of human agency, the spiritual attends "to the pull-forces of motives, which attract or draw forward—the language of spirituality is the vocabulary of 'ideals,' of 'hope.' Therapy may release *from* addiction; spirituality releases *for* life" (Kurtz and Ketcham 1992, 27).

Kurtz and Ketcham link the spirituality found in AA and other 12-step/ 12-tradition groups to ancient traditions that they refer to as the spirituality of imperfection. Human beings are viewed as neither totally depraved nor totally virtuous but as imperfect and flawed. The dark side of human experience is acknowledged and accepted; it is understood "that tragedy and despair are inherent in the experience of essentially imperfect beings." Spirituality is, in part, seeing the paradox that "it is only within our very imperfection that we can find the peace and serenity that is available to us" (Kurtz and Ketcham 1992, 28). The spirituality is a vision celebrating experience and enabling choice, not an ideology claiming to have found universal truth—a way of life, open-minded, questioning and capable of laughing at itself. This spirituality of imperfections fits with McKnight's community vision that I endorsed in chapter 1 and that is contrasted with the therapeutic and advocacy visions of society.

A HUMAN PERSON: REFLECTIVE, CONSCIOUS, SELF-DETERMINING
The person in Schmitz's (1986) formulation has free will to make choices, to choose good or bad, to reflect upon his or her actions and the consequences of them. Other phenomenological and social constructivist theories of social behavior assume that human beings are reflexive, that is, they have the capacity to think about and become aware of themselves and to make choices about their actions in relation to others and the social context (Berger and Luckmann 1967; Habermas 1971, 1981; G. Mead [1934] 1962; Wojtyla 1976, 1977). Many social theorists are interested in basic human capacities or ideal human capacities and do not distinguish levels or degrees of awareness of consciousness. The social conditions under which free will can operate most positively should be of major interest to theorists; the voluntary nature of self-help/

mutual aid provides a nurturing environment for the efficacious development of its positive aspects. Feminist social theorists consider the variation in awareness, consciousness, and self-determination of victims. Patricia Hill Collins, a black feminist theorist, views "victims" as those who have internalized the oppressive messages from powerful oppressors. They have taken the viewpoint of the oppressors and regard themselves as bad, culpable, "getting what they deserve" (Collins 1993). Many people entering self-help/mutual aid organizations feel and act like victims caught helplessly in oppressive situations; they feel, think and behave as if they have no viable choices.

Phenomenologists (Scheler 1954; Wojtyla 1976, 1977) have distinguished between two kinds of subjectivity—one which Max Scheler discussed involves the "emotionally conscious" individual, that is, a person who feels/thinks but does not necessarily connect his actions with their consequences; victims operate with this form of subjectivity, which I refer to as "reactivity." The second form of subjectivity as seen in the individual who takes responsibility for the consequences of his actions—in being conscious, she knows that her actions lead to certain consequences of which she is the author. Such subjectivity then leads to an understanding and acceptance of self-determination, that is, the person knows that his self or will determines his action. I label this second form of subjectivity "self-determination."

The distinction between reactivity and self-determination is crucial in mutual help. Many newcomers who are in pain or upset about their problem attend in a state of reactivity—that is, they feel like victims, they are conscious of their emotions but do not see themselves as the authors of their actions. As they experientially solve their problems within the group context, many people begin linking their actions to the consequences and start to accept their own self-determination; they become survivors or thrivors, emerging out of the victim stance.

Some thinkers such as Karol Wojtyla (1976, 1977) posit that with the acceptance of self-determination comes self-mastery, leading to self-possession or the gaining of a sense of one's self. Frank Riessman and David Carroll in their book *Redefining Self-Help: Policy and Practice* emphasize, in defining self-help, "self-determination" and "self-empowerment," "stressing the inner resources, whether in relation to the production of services or help or of governance and power" (1995, 3). In my terms, Riessman and Carroll's self-determination and self-empowerment correspond to the second phase of subjectivity (self-determination) in which the person links his actions with their consequences.

The path from victim to survivor or from reactivity to self-determination is a developmental learning process through intensive involvement in a self-help/mutual aid organization. The developmental process does not occur automatically; as the term "self-help" implies, an active willing effort on the part of the participant is needed to realize or manifest the potential gains. The learning occurs through a sharing of lived experience.

Lived Experience, Knowledge, and Authority

What is the nature of lived experience and its associated knowledge in relation to self-help/mutual aid organizations? The lived experience is primary in that it is firsthand and engages the senses of the person going through it (Reed 1996b). The experience is a process occurring over a period of time, not an event like attending a wedding or seeing a sunset. Grieving the death of a spouse or recovering from active alcoholism will be measured in years, not weeks or months.

John Dewey (1938), whose ideas on experience and learning by experience are so germane to this work, began with primary experience: things of "gross everyday experience" that are initially "fragmentary, casual, unregulated by purpose, full of frustrations and barriers" (Campbell 1995, 73). Dewey stressed both the undergoing of experience and the doing of experience as a matter of simultaneous doings and sufferings. Undergoing the experience can be confusing and inchoate if a person is new to the situation, has no framework of meaning within which to interpret it, or the situation is inherently ambiguous.

Experience is to be understood as a cumulative process of actions between a living person and her environment, a process that finds the person undergoing change in striving for control. Dewey maintains that experience is oriented toward future action and hope "by reaching forward into the unknown" (Campbell 1995, 71).

Dewey identified a secondary process of reflection by which the experience is turned into meaning and becomes meaningful—by focusing on one aspect after another, we gain some sense of the operation of the whole.

> Experiencing like breathing is a rhythm of intakings and outgivings . . .
> William James aptly compared the course of a conscious experience to
> the alternate flights and perchings of a bird. . . . Each resting place in
> experience is an undergoing in which is absorbed and taken home the
> consequences of prior doing, and, unless the doing is that of utter
> caprice or sheer routine, each doing carries in itself meaning that has
> been extracted and conserved. (Campbell 1995, 70–71)

The psychologist Edward Reed (1996a, 1996b) also has a useful formulation of experience. Reed develops an ecological psychology following James Gibson (1979) that considers how individuals and their behavior should be studied in terms of their relationship to their environment. His definition of primary experience is similar to that of Dewey in that it is what we can sense by hearing, seeing, sniffing, tasting, and touching for ourselves directly. Secondary experience is preprocessed or prepackaged experience, such as the photograph of the face rather than the living face one sees for oneself, or the information from the expert, television news, or the secondhand report.

Reed's ecological perspective posits that there are special features of the environment that are potential resources for people. Behavior and awareness, aspects of experience, are ways that organisms regulate their encounters with their environment. Reed's formulation implies that human beings are not necessarily aware of or acting upon the resources in front of them. This would include the person who thinks and behaves like a victim; such an individual frequently believes she has little or no choice in an environment that she interprets to be hostile and punishing.

Experience can be described either as a process or in terms of its content. Dewey writes that "'experience' is what James called a double-barrelled word. Like its congeners, life and history, it includes *what* men do and suffer, *what* they strive for, love, believe and endure, and also *how* men act and are acted upon, the ways in which they do and suffer, desire and enjoy, see, believe, imagine—in short, processes of *experiencing*" (Campbell 1995, 69).

Self-help/mutual aid organizations encompass the experiential knowledge of hundreds or even thousands of different conditions and predicaments. The sheer volume is staggering. For illustration, consider the content Marsha Schubert (1991) found in her study of a self-help group for parents of children who were both intellectually gifted and had learning disabilities. She followed the group over four years, surveyed attendees, and observed meetings in order to identify the experiential knowledge that developed. Schubert and Borkman (1994) classified the topical areas of experiential knowledge into eight analytically based categories; (1) understanding the nature and symptoms of the problem, (2) concerns about their own child's behavior and symptoms, (3) the impact on the family, (4) obtaining appropriate help for their children from the schools, (5) obtaining help from private sources, (6) providing practical help at home, (7) benefits received from the parent group, and (8) miscellaneous concerns, often unique situations faced by a family. Some categories, such as (1), (2), and (7), are common to all predicaments for which groups form. The specifics of categories (4) through (6), which involve getting appropriate help, would vary according to the predicament. Existential, spiritual, religious, and identity issues are common topics found in some predicaments for which groups form.[6]

My focus then is more on the process of experiential learning, rather than its content: the learning process by which the primary experience is thought about and reflected upon, the meanings applied to it, and the individual's dawning awareness of what he knows and that he knows that he knows.

Another illustration, showing that the process and the content of experiential knowledge are intertwined, comes from Alcoholics Anonymous, the most thoroughly researched self-help group. Experiential knowledge about active alcoholism is one part of the content; the knowledge of recovery using the 12-step/anonymous program is another part. The content of experiential knowledge is an integral part of the meaning perspective of AA. For example, alcoholism is defined as a progressive chronic disease that the individual is not responsible for having caused. The recovering individual, however, is responsible for arresting his disease by not drinking alcohol (or using other psychoactive drugs). Recovering alcoholics describe the content and process of their experiences of becoming an alcoholic with their "drunk-a-log," their story of their drinking years and the accompanying consequences: hangovers and blackouts, arrests for driving while intoxicated, lost jobs, broken marriages and lost friendships, and so forth. Their sobriety story tells the process of their recovery, of how they stopped drinking, what actions they have taken to stay sober, how their life has changed as a result of not drinking, and how they are interpreting and applying the 12 steps and other ideas for recovery in their daily life (Rudy 1986).

EXPERIENCE AS KNOWLEDGE

In contemporary life, knowledge is often equated with information that can be codified like a multiplication table or a data bank on a computer hard drive. We further tend to equate knowledge with intellectualized thought—that which can be articulated and expressed verbally or in written form.

The sociologist Alvin Gouldner makes a distinction between codifiable knowledge and knowledge as awareness, the latter applying to experience as knowledge. The pursuit of information conceives of the resultant knowledge as depersonalized—as a product that is found in a card file, library, or data bank.

> Such knowledge does not have to be recallable by a specific knower
> and, indeed, does not have to be in the mind of any person; all that
> need be known about it is its "location." Knowledge as information,
> then, is the attribute of a *culture* rather than of a person; its meaning,

> pursuit, and consequence are all depersonalized. Knowledge as
> awareness, however, is quite another matter, for it has no existence,
> apart from the persons that pursue and express it. Awareness is an
> attribute of persons, even though it is influenced by the location of
> these persons in specific cultures or in parts of a social structure. A
> culture may assist or hinder in attaining awareness, but a culture as
> such cannot be aware. (Gouldner 1993, 469)

Experiential knowledge is more "awareness" than it is information that can be captured and contained in a book, library, or computer file. Most experiential knowledge is transmitted through stories, often orally, and it is either difficult or undesirable to codify much of it in written form. Much of it is local and transitory—for example, how do I, Joe Jones, get through my first sober Christmas without drinking in Bethesda, Maryland, when I have two parties and three family gatherings to attend, where all that alcohol will be flowing?

> Knowing as awareness involves not a simple impersonal effort of
> segmented "role players," but a personalized effort by whole, embodied
> men. The character and quality of such knowing is molded not only
> by a man's technical skills or even by his "intelligence alone" but also
> by all he is and wants, his courage, passion no less than his objectivity.
> In the last analysis, if a man wants to change what he knows he must
> change how he lives. (Gouldner 1993, 469)

Following from the emphasis of experience as behavior and awareness, knowledge from experience can either result in awareness as described by Gouldner or remain simply at the level of unreflected behavior. Self-helpers describe knowing as involving bodily actions, not just intellectualized thought; action is highlighted and distinguished from awareness, understanding, or feeling. The intellectualized "head" knowledge is distinguished from the "gut level" knowledge associated with action, and it is knowledge-as-action that is important. The saying in 12-step programs that some people "talk the talk but don't walk the walk" refers to those who verbalize the intellectualized knowledge of what to do but whose behavior and awareness is not in keeping with it.

The idea that intellectual knowledge is inadequate to affect behavior is expressed by a recovering alcoholic in his forties who has been sober for twelve years:

> Although you learn something in an intellectual sense, a lot of what
> you learned intellectually has to be transferred to the gut, has to
> become part of the lifestyle. Sure, you can know that booze is going to
> kill you. But unless you're absolutely convinced it's going to kill you if

you drink again, you might go out and drink again. If you're playing a mind game with the whole game, it's just flat out not going to work. (Borkman 1979, 93)

In 12-step/anonymous programs the fact that action is the focus is also revealed in such slogans as "do the next right thing," "utilize, don't analyze," and "mood follows action." This focus on action or behavior regardless of one's feelings or thoughts needs to be emphasized as an important aspect in mutual aid, especially the 12-step/12-tradition groups; the short-term coping and long-term coping groups (cells 1 and 2 in table 1.1) are less likely to emphasize action. Action is based on implicit or tacit assumptions such as cause-and-effect relationships. Many philosophers and scientists have commented on the extent to which our knowledge-as-action is in fact implicit or tacit; Nancy Dixon (1994) quotes estimates that 90 percent of what we know-as-action is tacit.[7] These tacit assumptions underlying behavior need to become explicit in order to examine them in the process of making significant changes that will persist.

Public health has relied on the health belief model to understand the links among knowledge, attitude, and behavior. The assumption is that knowledge leads to attitude change which leads to behavior change; this is also referred to in the literature as "K-A-B." Prevention and health promotion programs are designed to change behavior based on this model. Thus a health education program will increase the viewer's knowledge of the harmful effects of secondhand smoke and the increased susceptibility to asthma, lung cancer, and other respiratory ailments of those exposed. The assumption is that the increased knowledge will change the viewer's attitude and then his behavior.

The K-A-B model deals in part with critical tacit assumptions that people make in relation to preventive or health promotive behaviors. For example, two assumptions contained in the health belief model are the perceived seriousness of the health problem and the perceived susceptibility of the individual to contracting it. Individuals who perceive a health problem as minor are unlikely to follow preventive health behavior; similarly, if an individual does not believe she is personally susceptible to lung cancer, this implicit attitude affects her health behavior.[8]

The reverse model is implied by experiential-social learning: "B-A-K," or changing behavior will lead to attitude or mood change which will increase one's knowledge. Lee Ann Kaskutas, Deborah Marsh, and Abigail Kohn (1998) found this model to be the basis for rehabilitating substance abusers of a self-help agency based on the 12-step/12-tradition principles of Alcoholics Anonymous that had been adapted to fit a nonprofit service agency. They compared two programs of the self-help agency with a hospital treatment program that

also taught the 12-steps and other AA principles to its patients. The professionally based hospital program taught the self-help/mutual aid recovery materials didactically, with the counselor-teacher lecturing to patients. In contrast,
in the self-help agency programs, the same 12-step principles were taught
through experientially based discussion sessions and through the participants'
everyday living, working, playing and interacting while in the program; the
recovering alcoholic/drug addict staff members shared their relevant experiences with participants.[9]

Implicit and tacit assumptions become explicit through narratives or
storytellings so that they can be examined in the cycle of experiential-social
learning. Through narratives or storytelling tacit assumptions can be revealed.

NARRATIVES OR STORIES AS MEANING

Self-help groups communicate through the use of stories or narratives. And
while the study of narratives has expanded beyond its earlier and well-known
use in the humanities to the behavioral and social sciences, narratives' value
for understanding self-help/mutual aid is still far from understood. Analysts
who study narrative emphasize that human experience is rendered meaningful through the narrative or storytelling mode (Bruner 1990; Polkinghorne
1988). The importance of narratives for creating and re-creating individual
and community identity is being examined; psychologists are studying narrative to understand such areas as memory, cognitive processes, identity, and
the process of psychotherapy; novices are learning about a new social world
from stories; Howard Brody (1987) has shown how reframing an illness, disease, or condition in positive terms can be healing to the sufferer. Stories function to convey experience, transform identity, and re-create alternative social
worlds. Julian Rappaport and his colleagues and students have led the research
on the use of narratives in self-help/mutual aid.[10]

Narratives are a way of ordering experience (framing), a way of "constructing" a world, categorizing events and people within it, and characterizing its
flow. A narrative contains a unique sequence of events, mental states, and
happenings involving human beings as the actors. A narrative is concrete.
Jerome Bruner, however, maintains that these aspects do not constitute meaning in and of themselves; the "meaning is given by their place in the overall
configuration of the sequence as a whole—its plot." Without framing, we
would "be lost in a murk of chaotic experience and probably would not have
survived as a species in any case" (1990, 43). The idea of "meaning perspective" as used in this book is somewhat analogous to the idea of framing as
Bruner uses it for narratives.[11]

Howard Brody, a humanistic physician, in *Stories of Sickness* (1987) makes distinctions similar to those of Bruner that contrast the storytelling mode of description and explanation with the biomedical discourse of science and medicine. Brody argues that medicine is a craft that involves the application of logical-scientific knowledge to a particular patient for restorative purposes (1987, 33). Medicine is a social activity grounded in ethical principles of healing and restoring patients. Unlike science, which is oriented toward developing universal laws or finding "truth," medicine applies scientific knowledge within its ethical, economic, and social context. "Stories are essential as a means of perceiving how scientific knowledge, in its generality, can be applied to individuals, in all their particularity. But recently the emphasis on the scientific features of medicine, to the neglect of its craftlike and moral dimensions, has taken a toll" (Brody 1987, 3). He argues that physicians devalue storytelling when they expect patients to restrict their litany of symptoms to those that will fit into the medical history.

Brody describes how we understand a human life through understanding a person's story. Four separable aspects are mutually interdependent: a human life conceived as a single entity from birth, through growth and middle age, to death; the human intelligibility of action; accountability for one's action; and the concept of personal identity. "One's action is truly one's *own*, for which one is responsible, because it appears in the narrative of one's life in an intelligible manner. The narrative serves to explain the connectedness of that action with one's other actions, motives, and desires. . . . But at the same time, personal responsibility presupposes that the person whom we are now holding responsible is the *same* person as the one who committed the act" (Brody 1987, 45).

Cheryl Mattingly (1991), like Brody, is interested in how practitioners can use storytelling to reflect upon their practice. She argues that storytelling and story analysis facilitate a kind of reflection that considers the ordinarily tacit assumptions and ideas that guide practice. "Stories point toward deep beliefs and assumptions that people often cannot tell in propositional or denotative form, the 'practical theories' and deeply held images that guide their actions" (Mattingly 1991, 236). In her work with occupational therapists, she found that the biomedical discourse allowed them to convey reasoning about the body, but storytelling allowed them to talk about how they helped patients live a disabled life. "Storytelling is an everyday way to make sense of or add sense to things that happen to us" (Mattingly 1991, 237).

The experiential-social learning process can be a reflective narrative process that is the equivalent of the reflective storytelling in a collective that Mattingly described among occupational therapists. The therapists were occupational peers doing the same kind of work. Each therapist interpreted what she saw on a videotape of a therapist working with a patient and described it to the others, which was the equivalent of a "circle of sharing." Among them, they had a variety of interpretations about the same situation, but they respected the others' views. They learned from the various perspectives, and learned that no single interpretation was "correct" or complete and adequate. They concluded that they could articulate more of the complexities, contingencies, and improvisational nature of doing their work through the storytelling mode than they could through an equivalent biomedical description and explanation. They saw more conflict in the video between what the patient wanted and what the occupational therapist wanted than in the biomedical discourse. The reflective storytelling revealed how they helped patients to adjust to a disability that the "chart talk" did not adequately reveal.

Self-help groups do the equivalent of reflecting upon their practice—which is the practice of living.

EXPERIENTIAL-SOCIAL LEARNING

The concept of experiential learning as used here has similarities with its counterpart in the field of education, except that here it refers to personal lived experience in "real life," not to simulations or constructed exercises used to simulate "real life." The field of adult education provides many conceptual schemes and ideas that match the realities of the learning process in self-help groups; this parallel, however, has not been integrated into the literature on self-help groups. Adult education and learning is a broader, more encompassing framework from which to view mutual help than that of "therapy" or professional services—the therapeutic vision. It is a framework that fits with the alternative community vision of society. The self-help collectivity then can be viewed as a learning space in which opportunities are created by and for the participants to solve problems, that is, to guide, model, and inform them of the group's framework for redefining and living their trouble and their identity in a meaningful, self-respectful manner.

Adult education emphasizes lifelong learning among adults (Cross 1988). The field cuts a broad swath that includes group therapy, training, classroom education, and experiential learning from life. Much of the adult education literature explicitly deals with voluntary situations, since adults are not mandated by law to go to school but choose to go (except for continuing education requirements in some occupations). The learner decides what he wants to learn, how much, where, and when; he learns at his own pace. The interest in learning on the part of adults is problem-oriented, practical, and for enrichment.

People enter any educational situation with a meaning perspective or worldview. Worldview refers to one's "assumptive world," or set of values, expectations, and images of oneself and others that are closely linked to one's emotions, feelings, and well-being. One's worldview guides one's behavior and perceptions (Kennedy and Humphreys 1994). Nancy Dixon (1994) uses the term "meaning structure" to denote the set of assumptions underlying one's worldview, and she emphasizes that most of our assumptions are implicit and therefore difficult to call to awareness.

The field of adult education emphasizes that an individual's worldview has to be taken into account in the teaching-learning process. Learning is seen as taking place in a wide variety of settings, including community settings, not just institutional ones. There is not the automatic assumption that only the teacher is a professional; many kinds of people can be the "teachers." Educational theory in this field includes the work of Paulo Freire and others who talk about consciousness raising and becoming empowered for advocacy as functions of education.[12]

A few contemporary theorists write about "experiential learning" in the tradition of John Dewey, Kurt Lewin, and others. David Kolb's *Experiential Learning: Experience as the Source of Learning and Development* (1984) reviews the contributions of Dewey, Lewin, Piaget, and others to our understanding of experiential learning. The twin components of concrete experience in the world followed by a reflective phase are found in all models. Kolb's analysis (1984, chap. 2) suggests that the models of experiential learning of Dewey, Lewin, and Piaget all had similar assumptions and propositions about learning:

Learning is best conceived as a process, not in terms of outcomes.
It is a continuous process grounded in experience.
The process requires the resolution of conflicts between dialetically
    opposed modes of adaptation to the world.
It is a holistic process of adaptation to the world.
It involves transactions between the person and the environment.
It is the process of creating knowledge.

Kolb applies experiential learning theory to social policy, lifelong learning and career development, experiential education, and curriculum development. His work is being used together with that of David Johnson and Frank Johnson (1997) in developing the cycle of experiential learning described in chapter 7.

The social learning theory of Albert Bandura (1977, 1986, 1993, 1995) has been suggested as applicable to self-help groups by Thomas Powell (1987), Miriam Stewart (1990a), Alfred Katz (1993), and Katz and Eugene Bender (1990). Other than identifying concepts from Bandura's social learning theory that are obviously applicable to self-help, little analysis of the applicability of these concepts to self-help/mutual aid organizations has been done.[13] Bandura's contributions to psychological theory and research on how individuals learn and change in a social context, especially how human agency is exercised through self-efficacy, are extensive. Self-efficacy refers to beliefs in one's capabilities to perform tasks, achieve goals, or control one's performance. Many research studies have been done linking self-efficacy with preventive health behaviors or changing unhealthy behaviors such as quitting smoking and stopping substance abuse (Bandura 1995).

Another set of concepts from Bandura that aid us in understanding self-help groups revolve around modeling, also referred to as imitative learning or vicarious learning—observing someone else's actions and learning from them without direct reinforcement. Modeling involves social comparison or the process of comparing one's performance or actions with that of another, either upward (I am not doing as well as Henry in controlling my temper in traffic jams) or downward (I am doing better than Ralph in learning to ask for help). Shelley Taylor (1995, 101) believes that the principle of modeling or learning that occurs by observing another person take an action without direct reinforcement is implicit in AA and other self-help groups for addictions; she suggests that "modeling may be one of the important mechanisms whereby group behavior–change approaches are often successful inasmuch as members of such groups can potentially observe and adopt each other's successful methods" (1995, 101). The concept of modeling is applied briefly to self-help groups in Chapter 7.

The sharing of experiences within the sharing circle of experiential peers results in collectively understood information about the pain, suffering, stigma, and personal negativity resulting from the common problem. What differentiates the sharing circle that becomes constructive self-help/mutual aid from one that remains the whining and complaining of the victim? If participants are motivated to find a way out of or through the problem with the group's help—that is, they are willing to engage in the self-help process within collective problem solving—they will persevere until they fashion a more constructive and life-enhancing way of living with their problem and regarding themselves in relation to it—they will create a new liberating meaning perspective.

LIBERATING MEANING PERSPECTIVES

People with a common problem in a self-help group share their experiences about the problem, which means identifying the natural phenomenology of developing the problem and its consequences in their lives, the ways they have been treated by family, friends, and others in society, their feelings about all these experiences, and so forth. These commonalities of experience carry pain and anguish, guilt, self-hate, and other negative thoughts and feelings. Members have internalized the meanings available from the larger society. In coming to the group, they want to problem-solve to find a less painful and negative way of dealing with their problem. But they need a liberating viewpoint about their problem and themselves in order to find a truly positive and self-respecting way of viewing themselves in relation to their problem.[14]

Sharing experiences helps to raise them to awareness, helps people see the commonalities (and also the differences) of what they have gone through, and is the basis for building a liberating epistemology. The new meaning perspective reinterprets their old understandings of what they went through, not attributing it totally to their inadequacies as a human being, for example, but partly to how they were treated by societal groups.

The meaning perspective of a group is usually distinctive in some ways from those of professionals specializing in their problem, or from the views of popular culture. Often the available perspectives from popular culture or from some professionals are stigmatizing, negative, and less than life enhancing. The voluntary sector provides opportunities in which people with a shared problem can create a social space and explore new and different ways of being with their problem than is otherwise available.

An example of the liberating meaning perspective of Alcoholics Anonymous and the way in which it is contrasted with the stigmatized societal label of alcoholic is given by Carole Cain (1991). She shows how learning the AA liberating meaning perspective through listening to stories and then learning to retell one's own story within the AA perspective was associated with identity change. She argues that the newcomer thinks of himself as a normal person who drinks before he comes to AA; AA, in effect, asks him to redefine his identity to that of an alcoholic who does not drink. A characteristic he entered with—an alcohol drinker—is left behind, and his "normal" self is jettisoned for the label alcoholic. One often hears in AA meetings that right before coming into AA individuals saw their behavior as "crazy"; some preferred a label of mental illness to alcoholism whereas others preferred the reverse.

Society's stigmatized label of the alcoholic has a different meaning within the subculture of recovery of AA, a point that is often lost on newcomers as well as observers. Observers often think that AA asks participants to degrade themselves when they identify themselves as alcoholics. Newcomers often feel the same way, which complicates the task of identification with the program. If the newcomer and the observer saw that the term "alcoholic" was not stigmatized but was a factual description of what was viewed as a chronic progressive condition within the confines of AA, they would not misinterpret the AA meaning perspective as is so often done. Similarly, the identity of a recovering alcoholic who practices the AA program is potentially constructive, life-enhancing, and joyful as described by the literature and long-term members.[15]

An important reason for the anonymity of AA is to provide protection to the participant from the negative perception of alcoholics found in society as well as protection from the stigmatizing responses of one's associates in the daily round of life. Within the AA culture, participants learn a liberating perspective: the alcoholic is relabeled a "recovering alcoholic"—a nondrinking person with a chronic progressive condition that can be arrested but not cured by maintaining sobriety and changing one's way of life.

The meaning perspective of a group is an important point of intersection with potential participants in the group. From the viewpoint of the individual with an unsettling predicament who is seeking help, a critical aspect of potential support—whether from a self-help/mutual aid group, a therapy group run by a professional, or a friend—is whether or not the other's meaning perspective is attractive to and compatible with his needs and worldview. The friend that trivializes the pain one feels about a divorce is not going to be sought out again for comfort; the relative who avoids the terminally ill cannot assist in the dying cancer patient's last weeks. But, as in the story of Wally, a divorcing Catholic, in the opening vignette, the people suffering pain like his were enough to connect him to the group for divorcing Catholics.[16]

From the standpoint of the organization, one can ask: does it have a well-developed and articulated meaning perspective on how to define and resolve the problem and a workable method for helping its members? Or is it a less-developed organization that is in process of fashioning a meaning perspective through the collective learning of its participants? AA, for example, has a well-developed meaning perspective that has not only been imitated by one hundred or more groups for other addictions and problems, but has become part of a culture of recovery in the United States. Other groups for newly recognized problems struggle to develop a meaning perspective that works for them. And although AA as a total organization has a well-developed meaning perspective, each specific AA group has to re-create its own liberating meaning perspective in interaction with its participants. How a group fashions and uses a meaning perspective is an issue that has not been addressed in the self-help group literature.

Self-Help/Mutual Aid in a Commons

Interesting but neglected questions can be asked by placing self-help/mutual aid within the context of the voluntary sector, which is distinct from the profit-making marketplace and the government. Self-help/mutual aid fits into the voluntary sector within the commons, a concept formulated by Roger Lohmann (1992). The commons is a public arena of action in the voluntary sector where "autonomous self-defining collectivities of voluntarily associating individuals" create and maintain their own social worlds of meanings, images, and sense of reality (Lohmann 1992). Lohmann's primary concern is with donative associations, organizations and groups engaged in volunteer labor, whether or not they are incorporated, recognized by the government, included in national data inventories, or made up of paid employees.

The commons as an ideal type has five defining characteristics: (1) participation is free and uncoerced; (2) participants share a common purpose (whether short or long term, minor or major); (3) participants have something in common, such as jointly held resources, a collection of precious objects (for example, a library), or a repertory of shared activities, skills, techniques; (4) participants have a sense of mutuality; and (5) social relations are characterized by fairness.

Self-help groups typically have all five characteristics of a commons. I examined the definition of self-help developed by the National Network of Mutual Help Centers, which represents self-help clearinghouses, and found a close correspondence between their definition and a commons' five characteristics (Borkman 1993).

Lohmann (1992) posited a number of premises about the commons based on research carried out on many kinds of voluntary associations. He contrasts the commons with profit-oriented economic activity, which many people assume motivates human activity. Lohmann points out that ignoring or explicitly rejecting the profit orientation constitutes a subjective attachment of meaning to the intangible social action characterizing self-help mutual aid. Of special interest here are the premises that apply to the essence of self-help/mutual aid, namely, the intangible nature of their social action, authenticity, and intrinsic value.

A premise of nonprofit-voluntary settings is authenticity. Individuals behave in such settings authentically: they are what they appear to be to knowledgeable others who are operating in the same environment. Individuals who seek to pursue their own political or monetary self-interest in the commons are behaving under false pretenses and are subject to penalty or expulsion. State charity fraud statutes seek to enforce such norms of authenticity. People who adopt a self-interested or profit-oriented posture at any time are assumed to remove themselves from the commons.

Intrinsic valuation refers to Lohmann's premise that commons should be evaluated on the basis of their own criteria, since they are autonomous social worlds whose values arise and develop from within it. The theory of the commons, according to Lohmann, refuses to give serious consideration to the prevailing proposal that efficiency, efficacy, typicality, consistency, and so on (that is, rational properties of practical activities) be assessed, recognized, categorized, or described by using a rule or standard outside of the actual settings where members have produced and used such qualities. This premise is consistent with those found in qualitative social research, participatory research, and symbolic interactionism.

Another feature of self-help/mutual aid is that individual members do much of the work of the collective to resolve the shared problem, that is, to achieve the common purpose. Self-helpers do not simply put in their money to buy shares or stock, hire someone else to do the work, and then reap the benefits. Their experiential knowledge and values about the shared problem are used in decision making about resolving the problem. If there are hired employees, they are in the minority and work under the direction of members. An example would be an informal food bank where neighbors pool their money and resources to buy food in bulk, save money, and get better-quality food. They do most of the work of organizing, collecting money, selecting food, and distributing it. If they hire someone, such as a driver to transport the food, that person is under their immediate direction.

The larger, more complex nonprofit organization with paid staff, say, a food cooperative with professional management whose employees are mostly hired, that characterizes much of the literature on nonprofit organizations falls outside the self-help/mutual aid commons. The cooperative is likely to be a legally incorporated nonprofit organization that competes in the marketplace with profit-making grocery stores. The "commons" definition allows one not only to consider crime watches, neighborhood groups, food cooperatives, and so on as mutual aid (rather than limiting self-help/mutual aid to the health and social service arenas) but also to distinguish those that are more in the nonprofit agency category from those in the commons.

THE PROS AND CONS OF THE COMMONS CONCEPT

Introducing the concept of the commons, an unfamiliar and relatively complex idea as the key descriptor of the social context and structure in which self-help mutual aid operates, has advantages and disadvantages. The commons covers a wide array of voluntary associations, including informal groups, clubs, membership organizations, and nonprofit organizations, as well as social movements, political parties, professional associations, networks, communities, and other activities such as conferences.

Although self-help researchers know there is extensive organizational diversity in self-help/mutual aid, the issue has not been adequately tackled. Some argue that many are organizations, not groups, and then call them all organizations. Others refer to them as groups, failing to distinguish local groups from national organizations with hundreds of local chapters. Benjamin Gidron and Mark Chesler (1994) view them as "communities of belief and interest," and their formulation identifies neglected functions that have been overlooked. But the fact remains that autonomous self-help/mutual aid covers an extensive range, from informal groups in living rooms to free-standing legally incorporated nonprofit organizations to complex national or international organizations with dozens of local chapters and thousands of members. In addition, there are networks connected through electronic bulletin boards or revolving around newsletters. Some have partial limited roles in the lives of their members; others are communities that provide alternative identities, cultures, and ways of life. The four-cell typology presented in Chapter 1, which describes four types of self-help/mutual aid commons, predicts that groups expecting long-term participation will be more likely to form communities than those with short-term participation.

Another conceptualization that can be compared with Lohmann's theory of commons is that of "community." Gidron and Chesler (1994), who applied the social science concept of community to self-help groups, noted three important social processes of communities: (1) a locus for the development of distinct cultures and individual identities; (2) a mechanism for providing social support to individuals, especially during times of crisis; and (3) an empowering mechanism for advocacy and participation in civil society (such as developing organizational skills and indigenous leadership).

Some might argue that the concept of community would be a preferable conceptual umbrella in which to locate self-help/mutual aid than the commons; certainly a broader framework is needed than considering them in relation to group therapy or as alternative human services. The idea of community encompasses many of self-help/mutual aid groups' essential characteristics, such as voluntary participation, mutuality, shared purpose, and broad functions, including the development of distinct cultures and identities. "Community" is a term, however, that has so many connotations, denotations, and usages that it has become limited. Community is also a concept that is difficult to compare with the concept group or organization, whereas commons by definition refers to all those structures as well as to activities.

The commons allows one to make comparisons across various types of groups, organizations, and networks or discuss seemingly disparate activities and structures at the same time.

We need a concept that encompasses all these forms and functions plus the social inventions we have not discovered yet. The concept should allow us to compare relevant aspects of self-help across organizational forms as well as to distinguish the variability in forms for other purposes. Much of self-help/ mutual aid would be excluded or inaccurately captured by the more conventional terms, such as self-help "groups," "organizations," or "communities." Lohmann's formulation of the commons accomplishes both of these objectives as well as others. Using the commons terminology locates self-help mutual aid squarely in the voluntary sector and directs our attention to other concepts and research findings that may be applicable to understanding mutual help.

The interdisciplinary field of research on voluntary action, philanthropy, and nonprofit organizations, sometimes referred to as the "third sector," undergirds this conceptualization of mutual help as an experiential learning commons. Many concepts and research findings from third sector research pertain to mutual help, but this body of knowledge has been infrequently and unsystematically applied to self-help/mutual aid. The social and institutional framework within which self-help groups operate is seldom considered, since the bulk of the literature on self-help/mutual aid is psychologically oriented research pointed toward the "therapeutic vision" of society.

The voluntary and nonprofit sector literature as a body of interdisciplinary research has at least a twenty-five-year-old history through a professional association of researchers and their journal. This literature is not without its problems and limitations. Studies of self-help groups are a minor and marginalized part of this literature, partly because of the focus on the publicly visible paid-staff nonprofits like hospitals, universities, and larger philanthropies that are discernible in directories of foundations or on tax rolls (Smith 1997a, b). The literature tends to be fragmented: discussions of paid-staff nonprofits that provide services under contract to governments constitute one literature; large philanthropies and foundations that dispense money are another portion of the literature. Quite separate is the study of informal and semiformal voluntary associations that are not on the IRS tax rolls and databases. Lohmann's concept of the commons was developed partly to address this gap, as a means of connecting the informal and semi-formal associations to the mainstream voluntary sector literature. The commons will be valuable for framing the entire range of self-help/mutual aid because it encompasses the widest array of voluntary structures, activities, and the principles of association within which self-help/mutual aid operates.[17]

Self-helpers assist one another without contract, money, or any explicit incentives—they are volunteering their time and energy. This volunteering may be quite different from the middle-class civil servant who volunteers two hours a week to help a nonprofit social service agency with its bookkeeping or who provides a one-time Saturday help to clear a flood-ravaged trail for a national park. Benjamin Gottlieb and Larry Peters (1991) separated people who attended self-help groups within a national sample of Canadian voluntary association participants; when they tried to differentiate the characteristics of self-helpers from those who attended other types of voluntary associations, however, they found them to be alike. More research that looks at self-helpers in relation to participants in other voluntary associations is needed to determine whether self-helpers are like other voluntary association participants and to explore who joins and who does not join self-help groups.

Another way in which the study of self-help/mutual aid within a voluntary commons framework will be useful is in considering diversity and variety in organizational forms; the voluntary sector acts as an incubator of organizational innovation. For example, early feminist groups for battered women or for health issues created innovative collaborative structures. AA, again, has developed a distinctive national-local organizational structure that retains control and autonomy at the level of local groups; the 12-step/12-tradition anonymous organization has persisted for over sixty years and has grown to become worldwide. Its distinctive organizational structure has not been well studied.

Finally, the voluntary sector approach is valuable for raising broader societal level questions about self-help/mutual aid. On a societal level, what is the impact of self-help/mutual aid organizations? How do they intersect with professionals and professionally based agencies? How do self-help/mutual aid groups as voluntary associations contribute to the creation of social capital? To the maintenance of a civil society and to democratic traditions?

McKnight's description of the "community vision" of public discourse (1995) provides an overview of this presentation of self-help/mutual aid in the commons and fits with the spirit of the civil society. Community is understood as a basic context for enabling people to contribute their strengths and gifts to others. The community has an overcapacity of associations, roles, and opportunities for work, recreation, friendship, support, and using political power. Those once labeled, exiled, treated, counseled, advised, or protected are incorporated into the community with the associations and network of relationships that utilize and celebrate their capabilities and gifts and compensate

for their fallibilities. McKnight recognizes community through six characteristics: (1) the capacity of persons emphasizes their strengths, not their limitations (the glass is half full); (2) collective effort is central: individuals work
together on projects that include the labeled and once treated; (3) informality marks associational life; relationships can be authentic and not managed;
(4) stories convey who people are, along with the history and identity of the
collectives; (5) celebration is a hallmark: one hears laughter and singing in
the halls, hears of parties and social events; and (6) tragedy also is part of the
communal life:

> The surest indication of the experience of community is the explicit
> common knowledge of tragedy, death, and suffering. The managed,
> ordered, technical vision embodied in professional and institutional
> systems leaves no space for tragedy; they are basically methods for
> production. Indeed, they are designed to deny the central dilemmas of
> life. Therefore, our managed systems gladly give communities the real
> dilemmas of the human condition. There is no competition here. To
> be in community is to be an active part of associations and self-help
> groups. To be in community is to be a part of ritual, lamentation, and
> celebration of our fallibility. (McKnight 1995, 171–172)

Chapter 3   The Societal Context

Y EARS AGO Peter Kropotkin ([1914] 1972) commented that mutual aid is ubiquitous and coterminous with human survival. While mutual aid is not surprising, its forms, the context in which it has evolved, including its interrelationships with other sectors of society, and the social processes involved are distinctive. Immigrants to the United States from Europe and Asia in the late 1800s and early 1900s pooled their resources and formed mutual benefit associations based on an exclusive racial, ethnic, or religious status. These associations maintained a group's cultural heritage while also obtaining health or burial insurance, loans, social life, and recreation (Katz and Bender 1976).

Contemporary self-help groups are significantly different in three respects. First, current groups usually form around a specialized problem. Second, current groups have common primary experience with a living problem as the basis of membership, regardless of the person's sex, age, racial, ethnic, or religious status. Third, emotional support is a central focus of the mutual aid characterizing most self-help groups whereas material aid seemed the primary focus of earlier mutual aid, emotional and social support being secondary.

The development of the self-help/mutual aid commons is typically attributed to the changes in society that led to the breakdown of the extended family, neighborhood, and other support networks, the increase in chronic diseases and social ills, and the inadequacies in the formal health and social services.[1] These explanations are important to understanding why self-help/mutual aid commons are sought as alternative support systems, but they do not explain why specific groups arose for each chronic disease, orphan disease, or social issues. Broad societal changes have modified the way and means by which people learn how to handle illness, death, birth, divorce, disease, and other life experiences.

Three Types of Learning Cultures

In one of her lesser-known books, *Culture and Commitment: A Study of the Generation Gap*, Margaret Mead (1970) describes the differences in how, what, and from whom people learn everyday knowledge and how they handle specialized problems. She distinguishes between three kinds of cultures: postfigurative, in which children learn primarily from their elders; cofigurative, in which adults and children both learn from their peers; and prefigurative, in which adults also learn from their children (see table 3.1). Mead's work provides a framework to examine historically how societal change within the twentieth century affects how, what, and from whom we learn about day-to-day living and other life issues such as transitions, suffering, illness, and death which are the content of the self-help/mutual aid commons.

Postfigurative cultures are illustrated by preindustrial societies or unchanging enclaves in which the pace of change is extremely slow. Older persons cannot imagine change or life being essentially different for the young from what they knew. The children learn from the elders the meanings of events and life passages, what their identity is, and how to live life. Content is unanalyzed and taken for granted. The United States in 1900 does not entirely fit Mead's criteria to qualify as a postfigurative society, but it exhibited more of the postfigurative characteristics than the United States in 1950, 1970, or today. In 1900, intergenerational authority was still largely intact. Grandparents were respected, and children acquiesced to the authority of their parents. Professional authority had not undermined people's confidence in thinking and deciding for themselves about many aspects of everyday life; many people had experiential authority about many aspects of their own lives.

Cofigurative cultures are those "in which the prevailing model for members of society is the behavior of their contemporaries" (M. Mead 1970, 25). In all cofigurative cultures the elders set the style and define the limits within which cofiguration occurs in the young.[2] It is expected, however, that the young especially will differ from their grandparents and parents. Cofiguration is likely to occur when the experiences of the young are radically different from those of their parents or grandparents. In the United States by 1950, there was a mix of greater professional authority that had developed with the rise and legitimation of professional experts and a much diminished authority on the part of the grandparent generation, but parents still exercised significant authority over their children. By 1960 cofiguration was the dominant

Table 3.1
Mead's Three Types of Culture

Name of culture	Characteristics	Examples
Postfigurative	Stable, unchanging society; old teach young.	Arapesh, 1925; Balinese until World War II; Amish
Cofigurative	Changing society. Learn from age-peers; expect children to be different from parents.	"Teenage culture" United States in 1960
Prefigurative	Change so rapid parental experience obsolete; young teach older generation.	United States 1980 to present

SOURCE: Adapted from material in Margaret Mead (1970).

cultural mode. Part of this involves the acceptance of breaks between generations and the expectation that each generation will experience a different kind of technological order.

Mead thought the "prefigurative" society was emerging in the United States by 1970. In this third kind of society children grow up in such a rapidly changing world that the knowledge and guidance of the previous generations does not apply extensively. Computers, space travel, nuclear bombs, global population growth, worldwide communication and transportation systems, genetic engineering, and the like have created a world so different that there is a complete break between generations. In the prefigurative culture, it is the young, not the parent or grandparent, who represent what is to come. "Now, as I see it, the development of prefigurative cultures will depend on the existence of a continuing dialogue in which the young, free to act on their own initiative, can lead their elders in the direction of the unknown. Then the older generations will have access to the new experiential knowledge, without which no meaningful plans can be made. It is only with the direct participation of the young, who have that knowledge, that we can build a viable future" (M. Mead 1970, 73). In the 1990s, the trends that Margaret Mead outlined in 1970 have continued. Children look less to their parents for guidance because many aspects of the world they experience is known more by them than by their parents.

POSTFIGURATIVE CULTURE: LEARNING FROM ELDERS
In 1900, learning parenting, occupational, and social skills were interwoven with everyday life. Children often witnessed birth and death, which usually

occurred at home. Sons and daughters were likely to follow in their same-sex parent's footsteps in terms of occupation and major activity. Stronger religious, moral, and value systems anchored the meanings of life transitions, disease, and death.

The rate of new information from science, the professions, and so on was comparatively little and slow. There were few paved roads, no radio or television, and many people lived spread apart or were new migrants to urban areas.

People had some exposure to books, magazines, newspapers, or travelers who gave lectures; but people learned mostly from their families and neighbors, especially intergenerationally and from their own experience. "Recipe knowledge" or folk knowledge was passed down from generation to generation about how to handle different troubles or resolve life's problems.

Advances in the biological sciences brought the germ theory of disease and other significant scientific changes in the late 1800s. These advances captured the public's imagination. More and more of the public saw the physicians as experts, turning to them for help even though there was little objective evidence that medicine had effective treatments for many diseases by the early 1900s.

In 1900 the life expectancy at birth was 46 years for males and 48 years for females. By 1950, it was 65.6 years for males and 71.1 years for females (U.S. Census Bureau 1975). Public health improvements (such as sewer systems and clean water supplies) and increases in the standard of living were primarily responsible for the drops in infant mortality and increased life expectancy (McKinlay and McKinlay 1994).

During the early 1900s, physicians gained increasing power, prestige, and acceptance as experts in diagnosing and treating disease; with this came an accompanying dependence of the layperson on professionals. People did not trust themselves to handle problems but sought professional help. The professions began to redefine problems and issues from their own vantage point. Sociologists refer to this as the "medicalization" of life problems in the areas of health and social issues. Issues were stripped of their natural meaning and redefined narrowly as technical medical diseases.[3] Pregnancy and childbirth, for example, were redefined from a natural life process to a medical condition.

As professionals strip diseases of their meanings or name previously unknown diseases, there is a void for the patient and his social network, especially regarding feelings about the impact of this condition on his identity and lifestyle. For example, science and technology developed the kidney dialysis equipment and procedures that allow many people with nonfunctioning kidneys to stay alive for years. This condition did not exist in 1940. Laypeople have no recipe knowledge about how it feels to be on kidney dialysis or how their lifestyle has to be changed to accommodate it. Professionals have little interest in helping people develop new meaning systems. Psychiatrists and psychologists might be interested in very specialized aspects of people's feelings, such as suicidal ideation, or in determining whether a patient's depression is physiologically induced by the procedure or is a reaction to the disease. But beyond specialized psychological problems, they tend not to be concerned about the everyday feelings and coping that dialysis patients and their families undergo.

It is the people undergoing the experience who must create the new meaning perspectives, which is more efficiently and workably done within a group context of experiential peers than as isolated individuals. The members have high personal stakes in evolving ways to have a positive productive life within the constraints of their new lifestyle. An important part of making sense of the chronic treatment involves its impact on their everyday life and the course of emotions before, during, and after dialysis—that is, is it normal to feel this at this point in the process? Is it okay to feel such and such? The dialysis "experiencers" and their families develop an "emotionscape" of the trajectory of emotions and feelings that is part of their experiential knowledge of the impact of dialysis treatment on their lives and ways to manage that. They develop a new meaning perspective.

COFIGURATIVE AND PREFIGURATIVE CULTURES: LEARNING FROM PEERS AND YOUTH

Since the 1970s, the United States has had a cofigurative and prefigurative culture in which individuals learn a great deal from their peers and from the younger generation. It is within this historical context that the rapid increase of self-help groups has occurred.

After World War II and increasingly from the 1960s through the 1980s, the pace of cultural and technological change quickened. The United States became an information society, professionals became dominant authorities, expanded forms of bureaucracy occurred (which George Ritzer [1993] calls McDonaldization), and diversity in diseases and life experiences increased. The term "information society" refers to the fact that more jobs are based on producing and distributing information and fewer on basic manufacturing, farming, or extraction of natural resources. The speed of change is breathtaking. Futurists talk about the length of time before what one learned in college becomes obsolete. The interval (five to fifteen years) is not long, depending on the occupation; people will have three, five, or seven careers over the course of a lifetime. As one's knowledge base becomes obsolete, one needs to be retrained. People start second careers rather than being retooled for the original one. Old recipe or folk information becomes obsolete, or simply yearned for as nostalgia.

A by-product of the rapid explosion of information is that many more diseases have been identified, social conditions defined, variety in lifestyles followed, and longer life spans made possible. People have an increasingly diverse set of life experiences. Self-help groups are creating new meaning perspectives that attend to the emotional and other needs of individuals. In that sense, self-help groups are a repository of experiential knowledge for society about coping successfully with highly specialized diseases, alternative lifestyles, and other newly emerging life problems that affect people across demographic categories.

People's recipe knowledge is more and more irrelevant. Many diseases and newly diagnosed conditions were unknown when they grew up. In fact, old age itself is a new social phenomena. With the extension of the lifespan, people contract chronic diseases on a scale previously unknown. For example, much of Alzheimer's disease is an occurrence of old age; it is more likely to strike people in their eighties than in their seventies, and more in their seventies than in their sixties.

Our informal social networks—families, co-workers, and neighbors—used to provide much of the recipe knowledge we needed to deal with specialized or infrequent life problems. Individuals could ask for and get help from their personal network. Now our social networks often do not contain the up-to-date information we need.

An associated issue is the way people determine that recipe knowledge is out-of-date and unhelpful. *Reader's Digest* (Summer 1992) has described folk ideas that are no longer true. For example, "do not go swimming immediately after eating" is now an outdated idea. Informal social networks are often selectively unhelpful—individuals have obsolete recipe knowledge but offer suggestions or comments to sufferers who find them unhelpful. Moreover, many professionals have only generalized or out-of-date knowledge about specialized conditions or situations. Self-help group members are often highly critical of professionals who imply they have specialized knowledge when in fact they are generalists about an issue and the self-helper knows more than they do (Schubert 1991). Within this context of rapidly increasing knowledge, the frequent obsolescence of knowledge, and the many new conditions and lifestyles for which one's social network is not prepared, many self-help groups for various diseases, social ills, and lifestyles have developed since the 1970s.

Other Interpretations of Contemporary Society

MCDONALDIZATION

One facet of the changing contemporary society is the process of McDonald-ization, a term coined by Ritzer (1993) as a metaphor for an expanded form of Weberian bureaucracy that has been increasingly developing. McDonaldization is "the process by which the principles of the fast-food restaurant are coming to dominate more and more sectors of American society as well as of the rest of the world" (Ritzer 1993, 1). This process maximizes efficiency, calculabil-ity, predictability, and control by substituting technology for human labor. Ritzer claims that the principles of McDonald's fast food service have been extended to most sectors of life, including work, health care, education, travel, leisure-time activities, dieting, politics, and the family. "McDonaldization has shown every sign of being an inexorable process as it sweeps through seem-ingly imperious institutions and parts of the world" (Ritzer 1993, 1). There is Jiffy-Lube, Toys R Us, U.S. News Today, H & R Block, Nutri-System, Pearle Vision Centers, Kampgrounds of America (KOA), Starbucks Coffee, McDentists, McDoctors, WalMart, and *croissanteries* in Paris.

The McDonald's fast food restaurant is attractive in a fast-paced mobile world with busy parents or one-parent families; people think they are receiv-ing good value for their money quickly and conveniently. However, with the rationality comes irrationality, similar to the irrationality of bureaucracy. Eat-ing or working in McDonald's is often dehumanizing, and genuine human con-tact is precluded. McDonaldization leads to homogenization and restricts creativity, expressiveness, and authentic human relationships. Ritzer is con-cerned about the future: "This critique holds that people have the potential to be far more thoughtful, skillful, creative and well-rounded than they now are, yet they are unable to express this potential because of the constraints of a [McDonaldized] world" (1993, 13).

McDonaldization is also occurring in health care in the United States. A vast expansion of profit-making corporations has occurred since 1965, when Congress funded Medicare and Medicaid. These profit-making corporations, whose ultimate loyalty is to the bottom line, attempt to rationalize and stream-line operations in order to hold down costs. Nonprofit health care organiza-tions are also being rationalized, emulating the practices of their for-profit cousins in order to compete and survive (Gray, 1991). Health reform is oc-curring at a rapid rate in local state governments and among health insur-ance companies despite inaction on the federal level. A major trend is to convert fee-for-service insurance to managed care. Managed care is an admin-istrative structure and set of rules that monitors provider performance and requires approval for certain procedures and treatments. Physicians and hospitals have lost autonomy to the managed care administration.

What is happening to patients? When consumers develop certain chronic conditions, the insurance company may not renew their policy to avoid responsibility for paying for their continued care. The provision of care within large bureaucratic hospitals or other rationalized facilities leaves patients feeling as if they are on an assembly line. Now they are pushed out of the hospital when the increasingly short time allowed by the insurance company is up. Patients can feel dehumanized when the nurses' faces come and go on each shift. Observers are already questioning what is happening to the quality of care when the emphasis is on the efficiency of operations and cost, not on the well-being of patients. And middle-class people can be bankrupted by an episode of catastrophic illness.

POSTMODERNISM

Postmodernism provides another set of interpretations about the meaning of the massive cultural, economic, and technological changes occurring in U.S. society as well as globally. Jean-François Lyotard considers the postmodern condition a result of the loss of credibility of the grand narrative of the nineteenth century and the decreasing legitimation of knowledge, including scientific knowledge (1993, 510). Charles Lemert summarizes Lyotard's ideas as "the ever-augmenting disappearance of the Center into a sea of relativism" (C. Lemert 1993, 492). Lemert also expressed this by writing that "no one seemed to agree on what, if anything, was real—and . . . no one had any final argument or wonderful story to tell on which people might agree" (1993, 493). Some postmodernists view a coherent sense of self as problematic since experience has become so fragmented, individuals feel powerless in the face of a globalizing world, and day-to-day life seems "empty as a result of the intrusion of abstract systems" (Giddens 1990).

POSTEMOTIONAL SOCIETY

Stjepan Mestrovic, in a book entitled *Postemotional Society* (1997), finds a parallel development in emotional expression to the emphasis on the abstracted, intellectualized rationality described by postmodernists. Mestrovic believes that emotions have lost their authenticity and have become abstracted and dead as a result of the process of rationalization of modern life. Using Ritzer's ideas of McDonaldization, he argues that public emotions, not just thoughts, have become abstracted and disconnected from reality. For example, Mestrovic describes "dead emotions" as the indignant anguish people now feel for what happened to their ancestors two hundred years ago. People may lose sight of the main point of an event in order to voice their upset; in the year-long O.J. Simpson murder trial, the fact that he was being tried for murder got lost by postemotionalists who argued that the trial was about whether African-Americans could get a fair trial in the racist justice system or by feminists decrying the lack of attention to O.J.'s pattern of abusive behavior to his wife before the murder. Disneyland or other theme parks provide another example, having been constructed and marketed by profit-making companies to manipulate visitors' emotions and convince them they are having a wonderful authentic emotional experience.

> Postmodernism has not triumphed over the question of authenticity. The daily diet of phoniness in postemotional societies cannot help but impact society profoundly at every level. On television talk shows, people disclose what seem to be their most intimate sexual secrets, but in the back of their minds the viewers know that these disclosures were made with the camera rolling. Inevitably, every disaster . . . brings the television journalist who protrudes a microphone into the face of the distraught victim and asks, 'How does it feel? to have had your son killed by a sniper's bullet, to have been raped . . . ' But something seems to be missing in these seemingly heartfelt disclosures of apparent authenticity. Part of what is missing is an authentic sense of community. (Mestrovic 1997, 97)

Mestrovic, like the self-help bashers, confuses emotional outpouring in public on the radio or television talk shows with the contained emotional expression within the closed and private self-help commons.

Mestrovic criticizes the tendency to resort to "therapy," which he describes as occurring from AA to psychotherapy, support groups, and abuse hotlines (1997, 87). He refers to the United States as the posttherapeutic society. He fails to distinguish, however, between the television talk shows and the intimacy of a self-help group meeting of experiential peers who bond in a sense of community. The self-help group is better suited to Anthony Giddens's (1990) idea that there are pockets of resistance to the postemotional society just as there are countervailing activities that counteract McDonaldization: the bed and breakfast, the gourmet restaurant, the specialized bookstore.

Mestrovic's pronouncements about postemotionalism seem to apply to some aspects of public life—manipulated emotions inherent in commercial theme parks, the media blitz over the death of Princess Diana, the television and radio talk shows. Individuals in these cases are responding to secondary experience in Edward Reed's terms—experiences that have been selected, processed, and managed by the media, professionals, and others (Reed 1996b). That individuals mimic the abstracted secondhand emotions "created" on the television screen is not surprising, as Mestrovic points out. In contrast with this secondhand experience is the firsthand lived experience of the self-helper, as found in the group for people who stutter in chapter 1 or Wally, facing divorce in his mid-forties, in chapter 2.

THE DENIGRATION OF PRIMARY EXPERIENCE

Edward Reed, whose ecological approach and work on the importance of primary experience are extensively used in this book, is highly critical of postmodernists (Reed 1996a, b). He notes: "The close of the twentieth century has brought on a deluge of near-apocalyptic rhetoric from intellectuals. Deconstruction and various other postmodern stances offer an assortment of metaphors of fragmentation, disconnection, and intellectual anomie. Theory and analysis are increasingly abandoned, replaced by verbal shards—some of precious beauty, others pointed and sharp" (1996b, 32).

Reed finds postmodernism flawed in part because of its denigration of primary experience, which has a long tradition in the history of Western philosophy. "Now in a final irony," he writes, "postmodernists like [Richard] Rorty reject the whole Cartesian worldview and insist that the philosophical ideals of truth and representation are myths" (Reed 1996b, 112). Reed thinks that such postmodernists come to the wrong conclusion; that the fact that representations cannot be true does not undermine "truth or the claim that we each genuinely experience our surroundings. Neither the representationalists nor the postmodernists have any concept of information or of exploratory activity, and therefore they have no understanding of how perception works" (1996b, 112). Instead, intellectuals and educators glorify abstraction and specialization over common sense and hands-on knowledge, become separated from all everyday experience except intellectual experience (1996b, 33), and make no place for firsthand experience in their theories, choosing to be blind to its importance (1996b, 112). These tendencies as well as the accompanying quest for certainty that can be pursued in intellectual thought but not in everyday firsthand experience contribute to what Reed describes as "why postmodernists revel in being couch potatoes" (1996b, 105).

Reed is concerned about the denigration of primary experience in our increasingly abstracted and rationalized society and believes that the lack of emphasis on primary experience in educational systems, among other reasons, is contributing to the current educational crisis. He also argues that the modern trends are damaging to our democratic system. "Increasingly, democracy has come to mean little more than a system in which we are given fragmented opportunities for registering isolated opinions. This reduces experience from an active, developmental process to, at best, a static cross section of points of view" (1996b, 145).

EMOTIONAL AID. Self-help/mutual aid commons emphasize emotional support and by default deemphasize material aid. Observers have not tried to explain this prevalent characteristic although they notice that in comparison with mutual aid of the immigrant and racial/ethnic groups in the early 1900s in the United States, little material aid is involved in current groups (Katz and Bender 1976; Wuthnow 1994). Is the explanation simply that the higher standard of living and favorable economic situation of the disproportionately middle-class individuals who participate in self-help/mutual aid obviate the need for material aid? This is unlikely. In 12-step groups like AA many are unemployed and in unfavorable economic situations, but these groups ask people to become self-supporting (this is a cornerstone of the traditions by which groups operate—the seventh tradition). Perhaps in reaction against the postemotional society that Mestrovic describes, self-help/mutual aid commons become havens for authentic nonpublic emotional expression.

A more plausible explanation is related to the fact that primary experience is the foundation of contemporary self-help/mutual aid commons in conjunction with the loosening of traditional support systems in a postemotional society. Within this context of the rapidly changing information society, McDonaldization, and postmodernistic ideas, countervailing trends occurred during the 1960s and later. Civil rights and other movements developed that challenged the tendencies developing in the information society and McDonaldization; they reflect what Anthony Giddens describes as "radicalised modernity" (1990).

RADICALISED MODERNITY

Giddens, a British sociologist, rejects the postmodern view that fragmentation, dissolution of truth, and splintering of self-identity characterize contemporary society. Instead he interprets the changing global situation in quite different terms that he refers to as "radicalised modernity": the reflexivity of the modern world allows individuals to create self-identity, and day-to-day life is "an active complex of reactions to abstract systems including appropriations as well as loss." Giddens argues for a dialectic of powerlessness and empowerment in terms of both action and experience (1990, 538). He sketches a phenomenology of modernity in terms of four dialectically related frameworks of experience: (1) intersection of familiarity and estrangement, (2) intersection of personal trust (intimacy) and impersonality, (3) intersection of abstract

systems and day-to-day knowledgeability, and (4) privatism and engagement—
intersection of pragmatic acceptance and activism (1990, 533). The traditional
bases of experience, such as one's identity and community being linked with
a stable geographical place, have dissolved. New forms of identity and community are evolving from the changing relationships individuals have to time
and place: self-help/mutual aid commons are prime examples of these new
forms of identity and community.

Self-help/mutual aid organizations certainly fit better with Giddens's idea
of "radicalised modernity" than the pronouncements of postmodernists. The
activity and advocacy, self-definition, empowerment, and creation of meaning perspectives that occur in self-help/mutual aid organizations resonate with
Giddens's radicalised modernity: individuals can reflexively reconstitute their
selves within an experiential-peer community. Groups and their members appropriate professional knowledge of their predicament and interpret it to fit
their day-to-day lives. In 12-step groups the dialectic of powerlessness and
empowerment has been developed extensively. Giddens's idea that the contemporary world provides opportunities for individuals and groups to evolve
new identities and situations applies in the next section, in which many social movements of the 1960s and later are described as countervailing influ-
ences to the supposedly McDonaldized, rationalized, and abstracted world of
the postmodernist "couch potatoes."

Countervailing Social Movements of the 1960s and 1970s

The civil and human rights movements of the 1960s and 1970s occurred in a
society in which experts were increasingly dominant, among other trends. The
civil rights movement for blacks and other minority racial and ethnic groups,
the anti–Vietnam War movement, and the women's movement spawned
changes that continue. Following these were other human rights movements
for people with physical and emotional disabilities, stigmatized people, consumers and others that seemed to draw energy from one another. These movements fought against legal discrimination, injustice, and inequality, often
through the courts or legislatures. These legal and social changes are well-
recognized aspects of civil rights for which the movements advocated change.
Less obvious, recognized, or understood were the "cultural rights" that evolved
as part of these movements. Cultural rights refers to the idea that groups, sub-
cultures, or social entities have the right to define themselves, and to name
themselves, to give voice to their experiences as valid. The slogan "Black is
beautiful" is one example. These trends are illustrative of Giddens's ideas regarding "radicalised modernity."

Participants who were brought together by their common problems also shared their personal experiences with one another—consciousness-raising groups among feminists are especially well known examples of this process. From sharing personal experiences in a group of experiential peers, they learned that they were struggling with common situations that evoked similar emotions and meanings in their lives. These stories of individuals being "in the world" are expressed in the subjective "language of the heart." People gained experiential authority. People empowered one another through their shared group reflections, encouragement, and hope. The process led to their conviction that they had experiential knowledge of their condition, although they did not give it a name. They became self-authorities. Their experiential authority gave them power among themselves to claim their cultural rights— the right to name themselves, to define their own values and reality—and to stand up against the dominant political forces that had previously defined them and their reality.

Cultural rights includes the capacity not only to name oneself but also to define one's identity.[4] For example, physically handicapped people say it is demeaning to refer to them as "confined" to a wheelchair. Instead they say that they "use" a wheelchair. Some groups of people who use wheelchairs refer to nonusers as TABs—the temporarily able-bodied—which captures the tenuousness of being physically whole. People who stutter do not want to be called stutterers because that typifies them by only one of many of their characteristics; they are first and foremost human beings with the same civil rights as everyone else. They have the right to take as much time as needed to make their request known in a public situation, regardless of the discomfort of fluent bystanders over their stuttering.

As an important by-product of the civil, human rights, and consumer movements of the 1960s and the 1970s, people with different diseases or social conditions realized that they could benefit from the mutual aid format that relied on personal experience rather than professional expertise. The consumer movement increased awareness of the rights of consumers. Dehumanizing treatment by physicians or bureaucracies in hospitals or agencies became more unacceptable. As groups developed stronger voices, their experiential authority as a collective increased. They challenged professionals to humanize their practices and to include them in the information loop and decision making.[5] This was the period when a host of self-help groups formed around conditions and life problems that had previously never been the focus of self-help groups. By the 1980s, the formation of a new self-help group signaled a new problem. Instead of relying on public opinion polls or experts to point out emerging social ills, the formation of new groups was a harbinger of unacceptable situations that needed to be ameliorated.

The experiential perspective, wisdom, and authority were also becoming recognized in society more generally. By the late 1980s the perspective and authority of people who had lived through various life experiences were recognized and validated in many ways. The 12-step recovery movement, widely known in popular culture, is the most generalized indication of the recognition of experiential authority. Television and radio talk shows that proliferated during the 1980s regularly began to use an experiential authority along with a professional authority. A person who was successfully managing her diabetes in daily life, for example, would appear on a talk show with a physician.

There is no agreed-upon name for experiential wisdom or authority among the public at large or among professionals. Experiential perspectives seem to be highly credible to many segments of the population, excluding professionals, scientists, and academics. These latter groups, however, have a vested interest in the dominance of professional knowledge since they are its possessors, many of them not understanding that experiential knowledge is not in competition with professional knowledge.

The influence of the women's movement and feminist theories and scholarship since the 1960s that validated the "subjective," the "experiential," and the focus on the private invisible sphere of everyday life has been substantial. Elayne Rapping (1997) maintains that the women's movement of the 1960s and 1970s, especially the consciousness-raising groups, is the main reason that so many women joined self-help groups in the 1980s. The values of the women's movement are similar to those of self-help in terms of emotional expression and the recognition that many relationship issues stem from family-of-origin difficulties. But according to Rapping, the 12-step movement is significantly different in a negative way from the women's movement. Unlike the women's movement, which focused on social action to change the causes of women's problems found in sexist and patriarchal societal institutions, the 12-step movement is focused inward, blaming women's troubles and addictions on disease. Rapping maintains that to define oneself in terms of illness is disempowering and diminishing. A backlash has occurred since the 1980s, and right-wing ideology has developed power in reaction to societal changes in the position of women and the family. Women in self-help groups are retreating from social action that could change their lives. Other analyses of the women's movement have shown the way in which social action connected to self-help/mutual aid commons has been directed toward changing and humanizing the often bureaucratic professional practices in hospitals and agencies; childbirth and women's special gynecological needs in particular have been modified owing to the advocacy of the women's movement.[6]

NEW IDENTITY SOCIAL MOVEMENTS

A recent analysis of contemporary social movements argues that the politically oriented social movements of the 1960s and earlier that focused on changing laws and regulations dealing with injustice, inequality, and discrimination—the type of social advocacy that Rapping implicitly discusses—are diminishing. Instead, today we have more culturally oriented social movements that deal with assertions of cultural rights, new social identities, and lifestyles. Analyses of these identity-oriented social movements began in Europe and are associated with theorists like Alberto Melucci (1985) and A. Touraine (1985); frequent examples are animal rights activists and environmentalists.

Melucci and Touraine argue that the new identity-oriented social movements deal with changes taking place in civil society disconnected from official politics and petitions against the state. The degree to which they take state power is not a measure of their success.

Touraine asserts that "the main political problems today deal directly with private life—fecundity and birth, reproduction and sexuality, illness and death" (1985, 779).

Melucci sees a glaring gap in our technocratic society: "no time or place for questions concerning individual destiny and choices, life, birth, death, love." Moreover, complex systems of modern society have eliminated from experience all that is not susceptible to verification and measurement, everything that belongs to the sacred. Because contemporary society is so complex and rationalized, the new social movements try to reincorporate more private, unmeasurable, and "sacred" dimensions into social discourse and social life (Melucci 1985, 35).

The new identity-oriented social movements are not expressed as traditional social movements in terms of large formalized advocacy organizations such as Ralph Nader's Public Citizen (McCarthy and Zald 1977), but are manifested in communities and networks of like-minded people cultivating new norms, values, and interpretations of reality. Melucci finds that social change is brought about through cultural channels—modernizing institutions, furnishing new elites, and renewing cultures, languages, and habits. He envisions contemporary movements as "a network of small groups submerged in everyday life which require a personal involvement in experiencing and practicing cultural innovation" (1985, 800). Melucci emphasizes the relationships between members in the movement and their submerged character. Members have the opportunity to test out and develop new cultural models, "changes in the system of meaning which are very often opposed to the dominant social codes . . . the medium, the movement itself as a new medium, is the message. As prophets without enchantment, contemporary movements practice in the present the change they are struggling for: to redefine the meaning of social action for the whole society" (1985, 801).

Kim Bloomfield (1994) has applied the new social movement theory to the case of Alcoholics Anonymous and argues that AA fits the condition of a partial social movement of the new identity-oriented type, rather than the traditional politically oriented movement to change laws within the context of government power. Drawing upon Ernest Kurtz's analysis "Why AA Works: The Intellectual Significance of AA" (1981), Bloomfield points to the challenges that the AA values and ideology make to Enlightment-inspired ideas of modernity, especially in the United States. The Enlightment-based ideas of increasing rationalization and control (which Ritzer documents so forcefully in his analysis of McDonaldization) are increasingly questionable in the postmodern "Age of Limits." The United States experienced signs of limits in the stock market crash of 1929, then in the Great Depression, World War II, the nuclear age, and the cold war. For example, as we understand that burning up the planet's fossil fuel pollutes the atmosphere, endangering life, we recognize the need for limits. "The fundamental modern endeavor, the very identity of modernity in modernity's own terms, [reveals] itself as inherently addictive: the idea of always striving harder for more and always being satisfied less and less" (E. Kurtz 1979, cited in Bloomfield 1994, 28). Kurtz sees the erosion of the efficacy of rationalization and control and the appearance of AA as part of a questioning of the meaning of rationalization and control. Alcoholism, for Kurtz, stands as a metaphor for the "Age of Limits," and he stresses that the AA ideology contains two essential ideas: the idea of the essential limitation of human beings, their finiteness and shared mutuality, and an awareness that humans are interdependent with others. The essential limitation refers to alcoholics' powerlessness to stop drinking alcohol through their own willpower and the need for a Higher Power who will assist them; thus they are essentially limited in the control they can exercise. But at the other extreme, they have the capacity to act, especially with the help of others; the answer to limitation is to band with others in shared mutuality.

Public and Private Spheres of Experience

Along with the information society, McDonaldization, and professional expertise that "medicalizes" natural events, there is what Peggy McIntosh calls a large "fault line" between this public world of institutions, professions, information, and work and the undervalued private aspects of everyday living: upkeep, maintenance, "subjective" feelings and the making and mending of social fabrics. McIntosh, at Wellesley's Center for Research on Women, provides a provocative and useful model of the public and private aspects of life (1983, 1990). Her model of society is an image of a broken pyramid (or mountain with peaks) with an invisible fault line near the middle. The faulted pyramid represents our institutions, culture and psyches as a whole.

The "top" realm, the vertical part of the pyramid or mountain, represents the most public aspect of the institutional life of society—within the government, corporations, professions, military, universities, churches, mass media, and so forth. For the individual, this is the realm of jobs and career, financial standing, social position, social, civic, or political activities or positions, and involves attempts to cultivate in oneself the functions of being right, being in control, working alone, being specialized, and being precise and exacting. Here exist a few elite functions, positions, and institutions considered to be "at the top," a larger number of middle positions, and a still larger number at the bottom. The values of these three layers of hierarchy involve competition, achievement, and success, winning or losing. Survival in this world is viewed as a matter of winning lest you lose; upward and downward mobility is a common preoccupation of individuals and institutions. Individuals are taught to see their institutions and themselves within this hierarchical "win lest you lose" framework.

The second realm is under the lateral fault line, which is invisible across the middle portion of the mountain or pyramid. It is the private realm of upkeep and maintenance, whether in public or in private life. It is the world of making and attending to relationships within both public and private life. The values and ethical system of this lateral world operate on the "principle that you work for the decent survival of all, and that this effort conduces to your own survival and your humanity as well" (McIntosh 1983, 15). Values are collaborative and cooperative, not competitive. "The idea of decent survival of all lies behind our friendships and our conversations and much of our daily life as we go about our ordinary business. Most of what we do is on this lateral plane of working for our own decent survival rather than 'getting ahead'" (McIntosh 1983, 15). This is the work behind the scenes and is usually assigned arbitrarily as women's work or that of other "lower-caste" people; it is the work of domestic upkeep and of the making of ties and relationships in all kinds of life.

McIntosh and others' distinction of public and private realms cuts across the sectors approach described in chapters 1 and 2. The government (first sector), business (second sector), and nonprofit (third sector) worlds exist in the public sphere in McIntosh's terms insofar as it is the world of work, politics, public media and the like in which people go to offices, wear career outfits, answer their telephone in a professional manner, and the like. The fourth sector of households and families operates in the public sphere when company visits, when the media show up at the door, at holidays to impress one's neighbors, or when they are otherwise on "public" display—their face to the world. The private realm refers to behind-the-scenes activity to prepare for the public or private realm.

Using McIntosh's imagery, we may understand self-help/mutual aid as involving the relational life below the lateral fault line. This is the realm of "subjectivity" and nonabstract, daily, practical lived experience. The experiential knowledge and understanding gained in the groups help people to maneuver in both public and private life. Self-help/mutual aid is, in one sense, a link between the relational world and the competitive dimensions of "objective" knowledge, professional services and public institutional hierarchies. Even when self-helpers use professional knowledge, they are likely to be translating and applying it to the practical everyday concrete level of their and others' lives.

The values and ethos that animate the relational world—collaboration, cooperation, helping everyone get by—are also the foundation values and the ethos of self-help (Riessman 1982) as a commons in the voluntary sector.

Other feminist writers such as Deborah Tannen use analogous images of two spheres of society—the male-dominated hierarchical world of politics, money, jobs and civic life, and the more invisible private sphere of everyday life that is cooperatively and relationship oriented. In *You Just Don't Understand: Women and Men in Conversation*, Tannen (1990) analyzes the conversational styles of the two spheres—the focus for the males on the language of status and independence in the "objective" public world and the emphasis for women on the language of relationships and intimacy in the "subjective" private world that they have been socialized to emphasize. Again, there is an analogy between the language of the "objective" public world, which includes the helping professions, and the language of the "subjective" private world, which includes the self-helper. The 12–step recovery movement has a highly distinctive and elaborate language for conversing in the private realm (Cavanaugh 1998) and for linking the "objective" world with the "subjective" worlds.

SELF-HELP GROUPS EDUCATE FOR THE PRIVATE SPHERE

Self-help groups are constructed social units with the objective of helping their members learn about and cope with a specialized issue or disease such as kidney dialysis, raising a mentally retarded child, or pregnancy and childbirth. The members are experiential peers who learn from one another. The units are open learning systems that obtain input from the larger society about their issue, especially from the professional experts and agencies that are regarded as authorities in that issue; thus, in McIntosh's terms, they link the "vertical" and the "lateral" worlds.

Self-help groups tend to be organized around the categories used by professionals, such as arthritis, heart disease, alcoholism, or the field of kidney diseases. The professional experts and accompanying government, private, and nonprofit agencies that specialize in specific fields dominate and control what is regarded as the legitimate knowledge and techniques of diagnosis, treatment, and control. Self-help groups, in questioning the adequacy and effectiveness of professional knowledge or practices, are experiential authorities with an alternative knowledge base and perspective. But they are not competing with professionals. Instead, they are concerned about the neglected, invisible relational world, the dehumanization that group members experience in the public sphere of health care and social agencies, and the negative social identities available to people like themselves. In a sense, they are specialized replacements for extended families and social networks that respect the humanity of the person. They are ideally suited for the contemporary situation—voluntary associations with minimal criteria of membership, nonhierarchical governance structures, and the values and ethos of the relational world. They are easy to join and easy to leave. The lateral world fosters the values and activities of mutual help: a place to be a whole human person instead of the one-dimensional façade required in the competitive world; a place to explore one's identity and what it means to be a human being; a space to develop intimate egalitarian relationships with others.

Self-help/mutual aid commons become "families of choice," friendship networks, and intentional communities for some self-helpers; these support networks substitute for the geographically based small town or neighborhood communities of the 1800s and early 1900s about which so many are nostalgic. Unfortunately, the extensive research on self-help groups yields little information about the frequency of these networks and communities, what functions they serve, or the patterns of involvement of members of groups; the psychologistic bias in research on self-help groups, which led to their examination in relationship to professionally based group therapy, fostered the assumption that the important things happening in a self-help group occurred during the convened meeting of the group. Accordingly, researchers focus on what happens in meetings and rarely ask questions about contacts members have outside of meetings, friendships that are formed, mutual aid done outside of meetings, and other activities such as social events held by the group. In contrast with this psychologistic bias is the opposite view that the purpose of self-help group meetings is to provide a convening time and place until a solid network of support and community has formed that obviates the need for specific designated meetings.

Robert Wuthnow, who studied the participation in small groups of a representative sample of American adults, found that 40 percent of Americans belong to "a small group that meets regularly and provides caring and support for those who participate in it" (1994, 45). On the one hand, he views the small group movement as a substitute for the disintegrated neighborhoods and communities, the smaller and scattered families, and networks of ties that supported individuals earlier in the century. On the other hand, he finds these newer groups to be superficial communities, because they provide emotional aid but not material aid, they are not as stable as geographical communities since members can voluntarily join and leave very easily, and they can easily disband. Wuthnow (1994) and Sally Helgesen (1998) worry that the homogeneity of small groups may hinder people from learning about diversity and co-existing with others with different views.

From research we know that the 12-step anonymous groups are likely to create extensive friendship networks, social and other activities, "families of choice," and communities. Some critics of AA, for example, think that too many recovering alcoholics restrict their social activities and friendships to fellow AAers; AA becomes a world within the world, a way of life populated by AA members (Kleist 1990). In Great Britain, David Robinson and Stuart Henry (1977) documented the way of life and community aspects of 12-step anonymous groups as well as other groups whose members' illness, disability, or condition permanently changed the way they could relate to the world.

One longitudinal study of a bereavement organization found that groups of newly widowed persons changed over the years; they began as members of sharing circles who did grief work together. As this phase diminished, groups developed intensive friendship and community networks and became social clubs, providing activities and events (Steinberg and Miles 1979). Wally, whose vignette opened chapter 2, relied on the group to provide social activities around holidays when he was sharing his children with his ex-wife, and found the woman who became his second wife in the self-help group for separated, divorced, and widowed Catholics which he attended for four and a half years.

Through studies and interviews, I have observed a wide range of relationships that self-helpers develop with people in their group. At one extreme is a self-identified alcoholic who has attended AA meetings for five years, maintained sobriety for most of that period, and believes in the AA program. However, she has never connected with anyone in AA for any length of time, has no sponsor or friends outside of meetings, and jumps from meeting to meeting without attending any regularly; she is very dissatisfied with her lack of friendships or a sponsor. At the other extreme is an alcoholic diagnosed as such by her psychotherapist who sent her to AA. Twenty years later, as a working professional with grown children and grandchildren, her social life and leisure-time activities are with her husband and family or with her AA friends, with rare exceptions.

Some people find self-help groups helpful in one life area and apply it as a generalized form of problem solving to other life areas. One example is the woman in Kansas I interviewed who helped initiate a self-help group for people with cancer and their families when her husband was diagnosed with cancer. After her husband died Barbara continued in the group, helping lead and provide guidance to newcomers. Some years later she remarried, but in time this marriage failed. Knowing the value of self-help groups, Barbara attended a group for divorcing people but was put off by the level of anger and hostility that dominated the conversation in meetings. She stopped attending the group. A friend of hers, Irene, whom she had met through the cancer group, attended the group for divorcing spouses; Barbara talked to Irene regularly about what she was learning in the divorce group and Barbara tried out some tips and ideas for coping with divorce that Irene had learned from the group. Her experience at that point was one step removed from self-help and mutual aid. In between are cases of people who attend a self-help group for a limited period of time, develop acquaintances while in the group that they may telephone outside the group, but whose ties with the group are broken within a short time (for example, an ostomy group).

The mutual help network is a learning community that involves the values, languages, and structures of the invisible lateral world. Groups help their members to obtain information, receive alternative perspectives, and create meaningful interpretations and stories of their experiences. Other functions of self-help/mutual aid commons are:

- to be a bridge by obtaining and transmitting up-to-date information from specialist professionals to the people who need it; this occurs especially in medically related groups.
- to assess, then counteract, useless, obsolete, or unworkable recipe knowledge from the member's social networks, from professionals, or from the mass media.
- to generate new meaning systems that link their illness experiences with their values, goals, and life stories.
- to become "families of choice" and communities for their members.

Chapter 4

Professionals, Agencies, and the Commons

The rhetoric, of almost mythic proportions, surrounding mutual help groups proclaims independence from professionals and formal caregiving institutions. The evidence may actually be different.

— Marie Killilea (1976, 81)

M ARIE KILLILEA'S 1976 statement still applies. The literature on self-help/mutual aid commons presents an exaggerated idea of the separation of self-help/mutual aid commons from professionals or care-giving agencies. Because researchers and observers have had a difficult time establishing member ownership as a distinguishing characteristic of self-help/mutual aid, we have been inclined to generate extreme rhetoric to prove our point, ignoring contrary evidence in the process. Ambiguity and sloppy thinking about the role of professionals and formal service agencies in relation to self-helpers and their groups still abound in the literature, in part because of a lack of understanding of power, authority, and interdependence.[1]

From the beginning of contemporary self-help/mutual aid commons in the 1930s, when Alcoholics Anonymous and Recovery, Inc., began to evolve, professionals and formal service agencies have been involved. The critical issue is the kind of involvement: providing access to resources or exerting authority to control the commons? In the cases of AA and Recovery, Inc., open-minded and friendly professionals facilitated access to resources—of legitimacy, information, potential members, and practical help—but did not try to control them. Leonard Borman (1979) describes the constructive role of professionals in providing aid during the early development of AA, Recovery, Inc., and other self-help/mutual aid commons. In contrast, an example of professionals taking control of groups is provided by Katz's early study of parents with handicapped children. Alfred Katz (1961) chronicled the evolution of four groups for parents of the handicapped over a five-year period; within several years two groups were taken over by professionals who exerted their authority in shaping the goals and operation of the increasingly bureaucratized organizations. Among other differences, the two groups that remained parent-controlled self-help organizations believed that parents possessed experiential knowledge about their children's condition and potential that professionals could not match (Katz 1961, 65).

The self-help/mutual aid commons cannot be independent in any literal sense from resources and institutions just as individuals and agencies are not literally independent but interdependent. All individuals and social units are resource dependent; the issue is who provides the resources and what is the source of control accompanying them?[2] Peter Lenrow and Rosemary Burch recognize the interdependence of professionals and their clients, including self-helpers. "In order to be effective in using their resources to serve the clients' interests," they write, "professionals must depend on the clients' active exercise of their own resources" (1981, 239). In addition to relying on the fees of clients, professionals need information from clients (a client resource) in order to diagnose or identify the problem and to develop an appropriate intervention, and also need the cooperation of clients in following the prescribed treatment or intervention in order to do a competent job. For example, the "therapeutic alliance" depends on the client's collaborative relationship with the therapist in psychotherapy (Davison and Neale 1996). Even more broadly, on a systems level, the work of professionals and agencies is facilitated if clients show up appropriately and if inappropriate clients do not clog the system. The situation of inappropriate clients is most starkly seen in hospital emergency rooms. Many people without health insurance or a regular source of care use emergency rooms indiscriminately, thereby tying up resources or resulting in ineffective and inefficient use of highly specialized and expensive resources. In contrast, many self-helpers become smart consumers and utilize formal service agencies more appropriately than their peers who are not in self-help groups.

The fact of diversity among professionals and service agencies in their reactions to the self-help/mutual aid commons as well as the interdependence between them is emerging as important but is far from being understood or accepted.

The year 1976 was the watershed in which publications on self-help groups flourished in social science journals. Until then a few articles on self-help groups appeared episodically in journals of various disciplines; but in 1976–1977 five special issues of journals or books devoted to self-help groups were published.[3]

The gold standard was professional group therapy and professional behavior, against which self-help groups were compared and measured. Researchers struggled to conceptualize similarities and differences. Self-helpers were
described as aprofessional to distinguish their form of helping from professional
(Gartner and Riessman 1977). The self-help methodology was referred to as
peer psychotherapy, and explicit comparisons were made to psychotherapy
groups (Hurvitz 1976; Lieberman and Borman 1976).

Self-help groups and members were seen as distrusting of professionals or
antiprofessional (Gartner and Riessman 1977). Few illustrations or other empirical
evidence were provided, making the basis of distrust or antiprofessionalism
unclear. My research led me to question this characterization. Instead, I wondered if self-helpers were becoming more confident of their experiential knowledge about their situation, thus questioning the professional more and thereby
appearing less deferent than the typical client. Such unfamiliar behavior on
the part of the client might easily be misinterpreted as antiprofessionalism.

In the early 1970s, I observed a group for people who stutter and saw them
learning to discriminate among workable and unworkable professional therapies based on their collective personal experiences. I saw their disillusionment
with speech therapists who claimed to be expert about stuttering therapies—
but in fact had no specialized knowledge about them; whose therapies worked
only in the rarefied atmosphere of the therapist's office, but not in everyday
life; who made promises that their speech therapy would permanently eliminate stuttering—but in fact the gains were short term; and who made other
claims about the benefits of their therapy that proved to be untrue.

On the other side of the equation, the self-helpers began to realize they
had unrealistic expectations about speech therapy: it was going to "cure" their
stuttering. As they learned, they lowered their expectations about what professional therapy could provide. They continued to obtain speech therapy but
for more focused and limited reasons. In other words, they became more discerning users of professional services.

Is this antiprofessionalism? No. Today we would refer to someone with
such nuanced and discriminating behavior as an activated patient or an empowered client. True antiprofessionalism is the rejection of professional treatment exhibited by the Psychiatric Survivors, who argue that their emotional
problems are exacerbated by the coercive treatment they received in mental
hospitals and from psychiatrists. Another antiprofessional self-help group in
the 1970s focused on the apricot derivative laetrile. Its members rejected their
physicians' advice and used laetrile as a cancer treatment even though its effectiveness was scientifically unproven and it was illegal.[4] The literature con-

tains more cases analogous to the group for people who stutter than to Psychiatric Survivor or laetrile groups.

The concept of self-help groups, including the idea that their members were experientially knowledgeable and wise about their condition, was not understood by the professionals writing about them in the early 1970s. In reality, self-helpers were pro-experiential knowledge—but professionals did not acknowledge or respect their special understandings. When self-helpers received little or no recognition or appreciation of their special understandings from professionals, they appeared to be antiprofessional.

As more evidence has accumulated since the 1970s, the consistent findings are that self-helpers do not substitute the self-help group for professional services, but use both professional services and mutual aid support. Moreover, they use formal services more appropriately. Mental health consumers in self-help or support groups are less likely to be rehospitalized or, if they are, have shorter hospital stays.[5] Thus self-helpers are not disgruntled or disaffected ex-clients (with the exception of some mentally ill patients previously under psychiatric care in mental hospitals). Self-help groups generate "smart patients" who have high standards for the professional services they selectively receive and can "teach" professionals much about the phenomenological experience of having the condition and learning to come to terms with it. Perhaps more important, self-help/mutual aid commons generate a less stigmatized social identity, a place in which to consider one's personhood, and for many a new quasi-family and community.

It is enlightening to deconstruct the assumptions underlying the self-helper (who was then referred to as a layperson) and the professional found in the social science literature of the 1970s. The literature dichotomized professionals versus "other people." "Others" included self-helpers, laypeople who rejected self-help groups, and the public in general, who were indiscriminately lumped together.[6] Others were vulnerable to illness, death, and misfortune. They were needy potential clients and patients and were seen as having few, if any, strengths or resources; many were stigmatized. The "odd man out" was a metaphor for the stigmatized and wounded deviants set apart from society that became the *Odd Man In* (the title of Edward Sagarin's 1969 book) when they joined a "huddle together" self-help group.

In contrast, professionals were assumed to be "put together," competent providers who did not suffer life's misfortunes or, if exposed to them, could resolve them through their own efforts. Professionals were seen as the expert providers who had the strength, knowledge, resources, and competence to provide for the lay clients.

Professionals were also seen in the 1970s as lone rangers who worked as solo practitioners. With the exception of some social workers and sociologists, in the literature researchers portrayed professionals as working alone. The government bureaus, health care institutions, and social service agencies that employ helping professionals were not discussed; the bodies of knowledge about the health care system, human services agencies, and government policy-making were invisible.

Legitimation of Self-Help/Mutual Aid in the 1980s

The legitimacy of self-help/mutual aid as autonomous, consumer-controlled healing groups that are distinctive from professionally run groups was strengthened by the national Workshop on Self-Help and Public Health, convened in 1987 by then Surgeon General Everett C. Koop. About 175 people attended the workshop, whose purpose was to determine how self-help/mutual aid could be linked with the formal health care system instead of remaining at its margins. Half of those invited were leaders and members of self-help groups or self-help resource centers. The other half were researchers, policymakers, health and human service professionals, or media experts sympathetic to the idea of autonomous member-owned self-help groups.

The concrete results of the workshop were disappointingly few and minor. Important, if not very visible, outcomes of the workshop have been the development of loose networks of self-help leaders, researchers, self-help resource center proponents, professional practitioners, and other observers. The directors and staff of self-help resource centers have developed two networks: the National Network of Mutual Help Centers and the International Network of Mutual Aid Centres. They hold yearly conferences, share resources such as software for information and referral systems, and provide support to one another. In addition, researchers at the workshop formed a loose network; from these researchers a Self-Help Interest Group was formed in the community psychology section of the American Psychological Association. The interest group is interdisciplinary and includes psychologists, social workers, sociologists, educational researchers, and nurses. It meets at the biennial conference of the section and communicates in between via the Internet. However, Surgeon General Koop accomplished the symbolic legitimation of self-help/mutual aid more than any material advancement of it. The mutual help movement continues to be primarily a voluntary effort, which may be to its long-term advantage.

Some consensus was reached at the workshop about the ways in which self-help/mutual aid is distinct from professionally controlled support groups.

Self-help groups were defined as "self-governing groups whose members share a common health concern and give each other emotional support and material aid, charge either no fee or only a small fee for membership, and place high value on experiential knowledge in the belief that it provides special understanding of a situation. In addition to providing mutual support for their members, such groups may also be involved in information, education, material aid, and social advocacy in their communities" (Surgeon General Workshop 1988, 5).

The workshop recommended: (1) self-help groups should not be viewed as substitutes for health and human services for which governments or professional agencies are responsible; (2) respectful, egalitarian relationships between self-help groups and the mainstream health and human service systems should be built; and (3) the participation of ethnic and racial minorities, low-income persons, and those with disabilities should be increased in self-help groups.

Researchers, practitioners, self-helpers, and others who accept the formulation of self-help groups as member-owned and member-governed entities are making both a value judgment and a technical decision about how to define such groups. My values include the acceptance and defense of self-help groups as autonomous self-governing entities (Borkman 1991). Other researchers, practitioners, and self-helpers are taking similar positions. An indication of this is an unusual effort to develop forums where professionals and self-helpers can consider and formulate ethical principles regarding the relationship between of professionals and self-helpers (Lavoie, Farquharson, and Kennedy 1994). The efforts of researchers, self-help resource center staff, and other professional advocates over the past decade have helped legitimate autonomous self-help/mutual aid commons and reduced the tendency to confuse autonomous self-help with professionally based support groups.

Thus in the late 1980s some open-minded professionals—researchers, practitioners in self-help resource centers, government policymakers, and others—became committed to promoting and preserving the autonomy and member-ownership of self-help/mutual aid organizations and to assist them by providing access to resources but not exerting authority over them.

THE LITERATURE IN THE 1990S

In the 1990s, professionals have begun to be humanized in the literature, and they are now assumed to be human beings susceptible to illness, bereavement, divorce, and addictions like everyone else. The expertise of professionals is not seen as omniscient; the need to question and improve professional services, if not taken for granted, is entertained seriously. The pioneering efforts of professionals who "came out of the closet" and revealed their humanity facilitated the change. A prime example is Fitzhugh Mullins, a medical doctor and cancer survivor who publicly revealed his struggles, worked for health promotion through a government agency, and led in developing a coalition of cancer survivors (Mullins 1992). Farquharson (1995) interviewed ten professionals who had transformed their professional paradigm partly through their own experiential knowledge of self-help groups; he refers to them as "maverick iconoclasts." Although Pulitzer Prize–winning journalist Nan Robertson violated the traditions of AA by breaking her anonymity, she spoke as an AA member in her influential book *Getting Better: Inside Alcoholics Anonymous* (1988).[7]

Similarly, in the 1990s the self-helper is no longer just a vulnerable and needy recipient of professional aid but also has strengths, resources, capabilities, and special knowledge to contribute to her own and her peers' recovery. Riessman's paradigm of human service (1990b) is an exemplar of this stance, which will be discussed in detail below. In the 1990s, research is beginning to take both/and stances rather than either/or stances toward considering professionals in self-help groups: there are dual status leaders who have both the common problem and professional training (Medvene, Wituk, and Luke, in press; Revenson and Cassel 1991).

Professionals and Agencies

DIVERSITY AMONG PROFESSIONALS AND AGENCIES

When one looks closely at the helping professions, one sees diversity within them. The concept of segments (Bucher 1962) within a profession is useful; a segment is a network of like-minded professionals who stake out certain claims and beliefs and whose practices are based on accepting and using them. Segments disagree with one another within a profession about diagnosis and treatment of the same disease. Many professions have segments with quite different ideas about the same disease or its treatment. For example, psychology includes community psychology and clinical psychology, within which are found cognitive behaviorist, psychodynamic, and family systems paradigms; there are also transpersonal, "new age" psychologists who incorporate spirituality into their paradigm and are not recognized by conventional academic psychology.[8]

Differences across professions are often great. For example, within mental health, psychiatrists as physicians have the state-granted authority to prescribe and dispense medications, whereas psychologists, despite doctoral-level degrees and credentials, are limited to "talking cures" or being supervised by the psychiatrist in terms of their patient's medication usage. Psychotherapists, licensed clinical social workers, and educational psychologists practice various schools of therapy and counseling.

The literature on self-help/mutual aid discusses professionals as if they were similar in their values, helping philosophy, and attitudes toward self-help/mutual aid. Research since the 1980s has shown that the diversity within a profession and across professions in relation to self-help/mutual aid is extensive. Farquharson (1995, 82) characterized three different professional perspectives: the exclusively professional point of view which views the professional as possessing *the* truth, excluding subjective or experiential ways of knowing; the human service practitioner, who sees self-help "merely as a useful addition to traditional practice"; and those who have a transformed view of their professional role and practice. In the last view "mutual aid is not merely an accessory but rather a concept that informs a new practice perspective" (82). For heuristic purposes, I differentiate among professionals in terms of their basic behavior and actions toward self-help/mutual aid as: open-minded, closed-minded, inconsistent, or indifferent.

Open-minded professionals or agencies are friendly and provide access to resources for self-help/mutual aid but do not exert authority to control them. These are the mavericks who have assisted in the formation of new self-help groups, such as Dr. Abraham Low (1950), who founded Recovery, Inc., the speech therapist who helped initiate the group for people who stutter described at the beginning of chapter 1, and others chronicled by Borman (1979). Those professionals who attended the surgeon general's workshop in 1987 or who subscribe to the principles that professionals should assist self-help groups to remain autonomous and to be treated with respect and dignity are other examples of open-minded professionals. Directors and staff of self-help resource centers are usually very friendly toward self-help/mutual aid and are among its most consistent and important advocates.

Closed-minded or unfriendly professionals and agencies are those who try to control self-help/mutual aid, deterring their autonomous member-owned nature, and fashion them in their own professional image as support groups. Inconsistent professionals are those who provide some resources but also exert authority in some way that restricts self-help groups' member-owned and autonomous nature, whether intended or not. The indifferent professionals are those uninterested in learning about self-help/mutual aid groups or who ignore them. For example, in the 1970s the group for people who stutter sent one hundred letters to speech therapists in the metropolitan area where they resided offering to tell the therapists about their group or offering other help to the therapists. Not one speech therapist answered their letter—that is indifference.

Some professional philosophies and ideologies are more compatible with the principles of self-help/mutual aid than others; this issue needs further research. In psychology, for example, the most obviously compatible is community psychology, which emphasizes applied health projects in neighborhoods, schools, and other community settings; it values collaborative relationships between researchers and people in the community, emphasizes people's strengths, and values empowerment. Many researchers who study self-help/mutual aid are community psychologists; some of them have risen above the narrow "therapeutic vision" to view self-help/mutual aid within a broad community context.[9]

This categorization of professionals can be useful as a heuristic device while more sophisticated ways of differentiating among professionals are developed. In addition to differentiating among professionals' stances toward self-help/mutual aid, we need to move beyond the professional as lone ranger (the truth is, of course, that the lone ranger was not alone at all: he had his horse Silver and his American Indian assistant Tonto).

Solo practitioner professionals or lone pioneers friendly to self-help/mutual aid are in a minority in comparison with the many professionals who are employed by government agencies, hospitals, clinics, and human service agencies. Many nonprofit hospitals, clinics, and agencies depend on government contracts or payments; their freedom of movement is affected by the strings attached by the payment source.[10] The extensive power and legitimated authority that government and professionally based agencies have is important to understand in order to appreciate the potentially vulnerable position of the smaller, less legitimated and weak self-help/mutual aid organizations in the commons.

SOURCES OF POWER, AUTHORITY, AND OWNERSHIP

Mainstream health and human service organizations are either government run or funded or controlled by professionals. Max Weber pointed to three sources of power in organizations: charismatic, or the force of personality as exhibited by Martin Luther King Jr., or Chuck Diedrich, founder of Synanon; traditional power, based on historical precedents as exhibited by the monarchy in England; and rational-legal power, based on one's position within the hierarchy of a bureaucracy. Weber pointed out that organizations institutionalize a source of power as the legitimate or binding authority. Since Weber's work in the early 1900s, Amitai Etzioni (1964) pointed out that professional expertise was an additional source of authority in contemporary organizations and situations. A fifth source of power and authority is the self-help group, as the bearer of experiential knowledge and authority. Some observers mistakenly look at who facilitates a meeting as an indication of power and ownership. The issue of whose power and authority pertains in an organization may not be readily apparent, but it can be answered by two important questions: Who and by whose authority can the group/organization be initiated, reconstituted, or disbanded? And who and with what authority can make and change the operating rules of the group/organization? When I describe the importance of self-help groups being autonomous and member-owned, I mean that members with experiential knowledge of the focal problem can initiate or disband the group and that they make and can change the operating rules of the group. Professionals can be "involved" with the group when involvement means such things as linking potential members with the group, providing resources at the group's request, speaking to the group at the request of the group, or being a regular member if they have the focal problem. When we define self-help/mutual aid as being member-owned groups, then, for example, Parents Anonymous is not, strictly speaking, a self-help/mutual aid group, because its rules require a professional coleader along with an experiential coleader of the group (Willen 1984).

There are in my estimation six areas of operation of the organization which are very important: defining who can be members, leaders, advisers/consultants; the agenda and social technology; what resources are used; and how the meaning perspective is developed. Questions can be asked about these six areas in order to ascertain whether self-helpers with experiential knowledge have the authority to make and change the rules or not:

1. Who and with what authority makes/changes rules about criteria for membership and applies criteria in selecting members?
2. Who and with what authority makes/changes criteria for leaders and applies the criteria in selecting leaders?
3. Who and with what authority develops/modifies the meaning perspective of the organization?
4. Who and with what authority decides on the agenda and social technology used in the group?
5. Who and with what authority makes/changes rules about what resources can be used by the organization? For example, are government grants/contracts, fee-for-service payments, donations, grants, fund-raising activities allowable or not?
6. Who and with what authority makes/changes rules about the use and limits of authority of advisors or consultants?

Relationships between Types of Self-Help and Agencies

Yeheskel Hasenfeld and Benjamin Gidron (1993) have systematically tackled the issue of potential relationships between self-help groups and human service organizations. Drawing on organizational theory, they show that four sets of variables influence the likelihood of interorganizational relationships: domain and mission, extent of dependence on external resources, service technology (the "meaning perspective" and social technology in my terms), and the kind of internal structure (especially degree of formalization and professional or experiential control). Competition and four kinds of cooperative relationships (referral, coordination, coalitions, and cooptation) are described, depending on the degree of interdependency, shared values, and structural compatibility between self-help groups and human service organizations.

The complex and abstract presentation includes propositions of conditions under which self-help groups and human service organizations are likely to compete or, if they cooperate, are likely to be minimally or more extensively involved with each other. Hasenfeld and Gidron formulate their ideas within the context of a modal self-help group which is described as having an informal structure, although the examples they give vary in degree of formalization and other characteristics. Their formulation is valuable in applying organizational theory to self-help groups.

Before the work of Hasenfeld and Gidron can be applied to real world cases, we need to categorize self-help groups in meaningful organizational terms and look at instances of how professionals, human service agencies, governments and foundations have facilitated the development of self-help groups and self-help resource centers. With Marsha Schubert, I developed a typology of self-help organizations that appears in adapted form in table 4.1 (Schubert and Borkman 1991). The typology pertains to local groups, the level at which support is given. If a self-help group is part of a national self-help organization, its relationship with its national organization is captured in the typology. The typology includes groups in which professionals have extensive control and addresses the issue of where professional groups leave off and self-help/mutual aid commons begin. Two variables were used to derive the typology: how dependent is the group on external resources, and who, with what kind of power, controls the group internally? Five types of groups were identified and validated empirically by comparison with real-world cases of groups. The types included unaffiliated local groups, federated groups who retained local autonomy vis-à-vis their self-help national organization, affiliated groups who were controlled by national levels of their own self-help organization, hybrid groups that had professional and experiential sources of authority, and managed groups controlled by professionals or agencies in which experiential

Table 4.1

Dimensions of Schubert/Borkman Typology of Self-Help Groups: Resource Dependence and Degree of Experiential Authority

External resource dependence	Sole experiential authority or shared authority	
	EXPERIENTIAL ONLY	SHARED AUTHORITY
Low	Local Unaffiliated Affiliated	Federated
Medium/High	Local Affiliated	Local Affiliated Hybrid (self-help agency)

SOURCE: Adapted from Schubert and Borkman (1991).

knowledge was subsidiary. In the typology the "affiliated" and "federated" types refer to self-help/mutual aid organizations. AA and other 12-step/12-tradition groups are examples of federated groups, since local groups are relatively autonomous from the national organization. Examples of the affiliated category are TOPS (Take Off Pounds Sensibly), Recovery, Inc., and Compassionate Friends, which require local chapters to abide by national policies in order to be affiliated. Parents Anonymous is an excellent example of the hybrid group: experiential and professional authority are shared sources of power and the organization is a hybrid in that sense. Professional leaders and their knowledge are required along with a peer leader to operate a local chapter. By the definition used here, Parents Anonymous is not strictly a self-help/mutual aid organization but is a quasi–self-help/mutual aid organization, or a hybrid. Another hybrid is the self-help agency, a new category that combines the rational-legal authority of the incorporated nonprofit organization as well as the experiential authority of the self-help group. The self-help agency receives government or other outside funding, provides services for fees, but its social technology is the self-help technology rather than professional interventions. Examples of self-help agencies include so-called social model substance abuse recovery programs, Centers for Independent Living for people with disabilities, and consumers/survivors of mental illness who run services.[11] Professionally run support groups are examples of managed groups.

It is important to reconsider several aspects of the typology. First, in the category of local groups, in addition to unaffiliated local groups, some local groups are allied to or receive resources from local human service agencies such as mental health associations or hospitals (see Remine, Rice, and Ross 1984). This instance was not covered by the original typology and accordingly a sixth type has been added: local affiliated group. The group for people who stutter described in chapter 1 began as a local group affiliated with a speech therapist who used his university position to obtain resources for the self-help group.

In addition, alliances and coalitions exist with organizations other than one's own national-level self-help organization; the typology did not allow for these cases. For example, the Alliance of Genetic Support Groups is a federation of autonomous self-help and support groups dealing with various genetic issues. Each group retains its autonomy but bands together in the alliance to pool resources and speak as a large entity on advocacy and public policy issues. The typology has been expanded to include these cases; thus, federated and affiliated now refer to any form of affiliation or federation, one's national-level self-help/mutual aid organization or an arrangement with human service agencies, foundations, or governments.

Once an organization is legally incorporated as a nonprofit organization, it has rational-legal power as a source of authority. When a position in the organization requires professional credentials and degrees, professional knowledge becomes a second source of authority. Legal incorporation as an organization represents a significant turning point. Rational-legal authority enters into decision making because: various procedures and rules are mandated by the state under the rules of incorporation; incorporation requires at least a semi-formal level of organization; and the organization is more likely to be a paid-staff nonprofit, which has been a critical point in the literature on nonprofits and voluntary action (see Smith 1997a, b). The self-help agency is a combination of a legally incorporated nonprofit service agency and the self-help/mutual aid organization; these agencies combine the positional authority of the rational-legal source derived from incorporated nonprofit status with experiential authority (Crawford 1997).

The Schubert/Borkman typology describes the sources of leadership for each type of organization, the likely role of professionals, and the extent to which experiential knowledge is relied upon to help members. As one moves from the unaffiliated local groups to the other end of the continuum, the primary reliance on experiential knowledge decreases and the use of rational-legal and professional authority increases.

The preoccupation with the professional as lone ranger has precluded systematic examination of the kinds of assistance and aid that governments, philanthropies, nonprofit human service agencies, hospitals, and other health and human service agencies have provided to self-help groups. There are instances of government encouragement for short-term projects such as hosting a conference on self-help/mutual aid in a field like genetics or mental illness or funding the publication of a resource guide. The state governments of New Jersey,

California, and New York supported the development of self-help resource centers in the 1980s, but California and New York withdrew assistance in the economic downturn at the beginning of the 1990s. Many stories have been told of grant proposals written and turned down for financial support for self-help resource centers from the federal and state governments.

The Community Support Program of the National Institute of Mental Health (NIMH) (recently reorganized as the Center for Mental Health Services) has supported self-help agencies of consumers (former mental patients) since the 1980s. They provide services especially to the homeless mentally ill. More recently the Community Support Program funded resource centers to assist other self-help consumer agencies. Following the success of these self-help agencies, a number of states have begun funding consumer-run agencies for services to the mentally ill.

Nonprofit health foundations or professional associations such as mental health associations, the American Cancer Society, and the American Heart Association assist and sponsor initiatives and projects related to self-help, but there is no systematic research on the extent of this aid, the conditions under which the aid is given, and related issues. The American Cancer Society assists groups for breast cancer (Reach to Recovery), ostomies, and laryngectomies, but what is the relationship of the American Cancer Society, a nonprofit professional association (of physicians), to the groups that it sponsors? Health foundations have funded projects for self-help resource centers in the United States and Canada; the Canadian federal government has been more involved in promoting self-help/mutual aid resource centers than the United States.[12]

When systematic research is done across various sectors of health and human services, I predict that investigators will find that many governments, foundations, and nonprofit organizations have assisted extensively in the initiation and development of self-help/mutual aid organizations. They also may have set up their own parallel agency-controlled hybrid or managed groups. When professionals develop and facilitate managed groups, they are quite different from self-help/mutual aid in the commons.

Self-Help/Mutual Aid versus Professionally Run Groups

The terminological confusion of using "support group" as a generic term (as does the public) or reserving it for professionally owned groups (as do many researchers) blurs the differences between the two. A comparison of self-help/mutual aid and professionally run support groups can be made by applying the six criteria of authority and ownership of an organization. In addition, the differences between the two types of groups will be illuminated by examining professionally facilitated support groups in terms of the criteria of the commons.

When one examines the characteristics of a professionally based support group with reference to the six criteria of authority and ownership, one sees that professionals, acting alone or as representatives of their agencies, set the criteria for members and for leaders, select the members and leaders (which might include an experientially knowledgeable member as coleader), set the agenda (decide how often and where to meet), choose the social technology (the content of meetings—lectures, peer sharing, and so on), decide on the resources, meaning perspective, and advisers/consultants to be used or not (see L. Kurtz 1997; Schopler and Galinsky 1995). Control of the meaning perspective can be done by restricting topics of conversation, such as not allowing talk on spirituality or of certain reading material, by encouraging topics such as emphasizing medically based measures of functioning, or by inviting certain professional speakers.

To further understand how the professionally controlled support group differs from the self-help/mutual aid commons, consider the characteristics of the support group and how these fit with the requirements for the commons.

Support groups are essentially professionally or agency controlled groups of people who have the same condition or predicament. The groups are constituted to provide information and support to the members and are member-centered in the sense that participants are experiential peers and their common experiences are used at least partially as the basis of support. Criteria for membership may include being a client of the sponsoring agency (L. Kurtz 1997). Leaders may share authority with members, but their legitimacy "tends to be based on training and expertise as group facilitators" (Schopler and Galinsky 1995, 4). The intervention technology of support groups tends to vary from open discussion to more structured sessions that help members with understanding, problem solving, and coping abilities but usually without an advocacy function. Support groups are often time-limited, lasting a set number of weeks.

To briefly review major characteristics of the commons, autonomy of action is critical in the sense that "actors in the commons are capable of acting independently and exercising both individual and group self-control. . . . The ability to act with others to create and sustain an autonomous social world is one of the most fundamental characteristics of nonprofit and voluntary action" (Lohmann 1992, 53).

Since professionals have government-mandated licenses and monopolies to diagnose, treat, and practice medical, nursing, social work or counseling and therapy, they are operating under the aegis of the government and the marketplace. Thus, to have an autonomous social world separate from the government (first sector) and market (second sector), one would *not* have a group controlled by professionals or bureaucrats or have a meaning perspective that was primarily based on professional paradigms.

Support groups may also be evaluated in light of the five characteristics of the commons described in chapter 2. (Autonomy of action is the natural result of these five characteristics.)

1. Participation in a commons is free and uncoerced. Attendance at self-help/mutual aid groups is not based on money or contract (the marketplace) or state coercion (such as persons convicted for drunk driving who are sentenced to a treatment center). The participant would have to be free to choose to attend meetings or other activities of the group and not have an actual or implied contract that specified rules of attendance. Support groups, in contrast, usually operate with an actual or implied contract between the participant, as client, and the agency or professional sponsoring the support group regarding the purpose of the group, the expectations for client's participation in the group, and the fees or form of payment, if applicable.

2. Participants in a commons share a common purpose. A shared purpose may also be a characteristic of a support group. The clients of a professional are likely to be told the purpose of the support group they are invited or required to attend. If they have the choice of attending or not, they may attend because they agree with its purpose. The dynamics of attending a group whose purpose was decided by a professional to whom you are subordinate as a client are different, however, than voluntarily attending a meeting and negotiating the purpose of the group with egalitarian peers.

3. Participants in a commons must jointly own something such as resources, a collection of precious objects, or a repertory of shared actions. A meaning perspective that members create and enact is usually a repertory of shared actions rather than jointly owned resources. Monetary resources are minimal since most groups operate with minimal financial resources. Professionals in a support group indirectly "own" the financial resources, which are attached to the agency or sponsoring organization. If professionals control the meaning perspective used in the group, it is then professionally based, not owned by the participants.

A repertory of shared actions found in a common language or methodology such as the 12 steps of AA and other 12-tradition groups could be owned by the participants rather than provided by professionals. Professionals however, can and often do appropriate self-help methodologies, as is often done with the 12 steps of AA. If a professional treatment program appropriates the 12 steps of AA and "requires" patients to complete certain steps in a certain

manner, then the professionals have changed the context of the social technology; it is not owned by the patients since their progress in treatment is
contingent upon completing the steps in the manner and time required by
the staff rather than the self-paced learning found in the AA commons (see
Kaskutas, Marsh, and Kohn 1998).

There are support groups run by open-minded and friendly professionals
who are committed to groups' becoming member-owned and developing their
own meaning perspective; the professional gradually phases out control and
takes a back-seat consultant position (L. Kurtz 1997, chap. 6). Judy Wilson
in England also describes the professional phase-out approach.[13]

4. A sense of mutuality refers to commons participants choosing to aid
and support one another in a reciprocal manner. Further, participants can
evolve friendships or various elaborated helping relationships as they wish.
Mutuality also implies that each participant chooses the level of involvement
and commitment he or she wants to have, which can vary over time. In order to have such mutual supportive relationships and friendships, the group
atmosphere and norms allow or encourage participants to respond to and help
one another as they wish both inside scheduled meetings and other activities
and outside of them in the rest of their life. Mutuality implies a milieu in which
helping relationships and friendships can evolve, depending upon the personal
characteristics and "chemistry" of participants. It implies that participants have
access to information about one another that allows them to make personal
contact, by telephone, mail, or electronic mail if they choose. In contrast, support groups often implicitly discourage or do not actively encourage participants to have relationships outside of scheduled activities of the group. For
example, telephone lists may not be passed around, or opportunities for people
to chat informally and get acquainted may not be available or be shortened,
thereby cutting off opportunities for friendships to develop or for helping relationships to blossom.

5. For commons social relations to be characterized by fairness or justice
as a political concern implies that the governance be democratic and that all
members have a voice in the governing of the group either directly or through
the election of representatives. Governance involves the important issues of
capacity to terminate or initiate the group and to make and change the operating rules of the group. A member-owned self-help group that shared leadership or elected officers would qualify as having social relations of fairness or
justice. A professionally owned support group in which professional leaders
led and made decisions about governance would not qualify for the commons.
Another aspect concerns the equal and fair chance that all participants have
to share their story; a circle of sharing is structurally more conducive to equal

opportunity than a lecture situation in which the expert is in front and the audience is in rows facing the lecturer. In the lecture situation, the audience may be selectively called upon to talk, and the dynamics are very different than the circle of sharing.

In summary, professionally controlled support groups are unlikely to become commons because the requirements for creating autonomous social action and controlling their own operation are rarely met. Specifically, of the five aspects of the commons, a shared purpose would most likely be met, and secondarily, mutuality of relationships is likely to occur to some extent, especially within the context of scheduled activities such as meetings. The other aspects of a commons are less likely or unlikely: fair or just (democratic) governance of the group, owning a shared repertory, and free and uncoerced participation.

Under some conditions a support group buttressed by professional knowledge and skills seems to be more appropriate than a member-owned group. If the potential members are very damaged psychologically or physically weak, vulnerable, or fragile, they are likely to need skilled professional help both in the social technology of intervening in the group and in maintenance of the organization. Or, in the case of people who stutter, the professional initially helped with organizational issues because no one had any experience in developing or running an organization. Furthermore, if the condition is short term and participants cycle through in a few months and then resume their regular life, the group may need professional assistance in maintaining the organization; these are the cell 1 short-term coping groups in the typology of four kinds of groups described in chapter 1. Professionals may be needed in support groups such as these for people recovering from strokes, who, with their spouses, are the vulnerable elderly; they may barely have the energy or motivation to participate in the group. Only the professional's maintenance will keep the group going. Parents in Parents Anonymous, who have abused or are at risk of abusing their children, are frequently from abusive families themselves and are likely to need professional assistance in the beginning.[14]

Whether some categories of people with physical illnesses or disabilities need professional assistance with a support group is problematic, however, since each case needs to be evaluated on its own terms. Closed-minded professionals, for example, are likely to assume that clients need help, which is not always the case. For example, many professionals may assume that the previously hospitalized mentally ill lack the capacity to support themselves and one another and to maintain an organization. However, many consumer/survivors of mental hospitalization are now running self-help agencies funded by state and local governments and providing services to their peers. Similarly, breast cancer and ovarian cancer patients undergoing chemotherapy in a hospital may appropriately participate in a hospital-convened support group run by a social worker. However, cancer survivors after their treatment often run their own self-help groups or agency; SHARE, in New York City, is an example (Miller 1988).

Professionals talk about a continuum of treatment for alcoholism or drug treatment, or for chronic illnesses such as diabetes, hypertension, or mental illness. Usually the continuum of care refers to professionally based services from treatment for acute conditions through rehabilitation and preventive activities for relapse or recurrence. Professionals are most likely to be needed at the acute phases of initial treatment. As clients gain strength, self-knowledge, and capacity, the professional can begin to share the responsibility with clients. Clients can become prosumers who provide help to their peers while still receiving support themselves. The continuum of care needs to include the self-help/mutual aid commons.

Careers for experientialists, people with a problem who have successfully recovered from it, become dual-status professionals with experiential and professional knowledge: the ostomy nurse specialist who has an ostomy herself; the previously hospitalized, now recovering person with bipolar disorder who becomes a social worker (Hatfield and Lefley 1993). In some systems, dual-status professionals are not allowed; in the Netherlands in 1972 while studying a self-help group for people who stutter, I found that people who stutter were not allowed to become speech therapists, a situation that did not obtain in the United States.

The Dominance of the Human Services Paradigm in the 1990s

By the 1990s the idea of self-help groups as alternative human services prevailed in the professional literature: the therapeutic vision was here.[15] Frank Riessman's article "Restructuring Help: A Human Service Paradigm for the 1990s" (1990b) is an excellent statement of this paradigm. Riessman focuses on the helping process, contrasting the traditional professional model with the prosumer model in which the helper and helped roles are interchangeable and one individual fills both. In the professional model there is a hierarchical and asymmetrical relationship between the professional helper and the client who receives help. The status differences are based upon the supposed expertise of the professional, grounded in his training, education, and knowledge. Rewards accrue to the helper, while receiving help can be regarded as stigmatizing and demeaning. Help is a commodity to be bought, sold, marketed, and promoted.

Riessman's article is especially useful because he articulates the alternative prosumer model that applies to self-help groups and related phenomena like peer tutoring and self-care. In contrast to the professional model, in the prosumer model the helping process is restructured. Peers in a basically symmetrical, egalitarian relationship both receive and give help. Receiving help is destigmatized. The benefits of giving help accrue to all rather than being limited to the higher-status professional helper. As expressed in Riessman's well-known "helper therapy principle" (1965), giving help thus aids the giver as well as the receiver. Help is not a commodity but a "gift" that is freely given and reciprocal (Medvene 1984).

On the one hand Riessman faithfully represents important facets of self-help—the dual helping-receiving role—but, on the other hand, he frames it narrowly in comparison with the professional-client relationship. The relationships between self-help groups and professional agencies are ignored. He calls the helping relationship the "human service paradigm" and, like other observers of self-help, leaves out the cultural and broader institutional contexts in which it operates.

Riessman's and other versions of the human service paradigm have become metaphors that shape our thinking and observations (Lakoff and Johnson 1980). Using metaphors as such is not problematic, except when one has a significantly different phenomenon and unwittingly assumes that the operating paradigm covers it.[16] The process of comparing self-help groups with the human service delivery system or its components highlights some aspects of self-help groups, such as the helping relationship; however, it ignores other aspects, especially informal relationships and community, the voluntary components, the way that problems are defined and resolved, and the broader context.

We need a new metaparadigm of self-help/mutual aid that is a level of abstraction above the professional helping–prosumer helping contrast that Riessman dissected. Beyond helping and receiving help, self-help/mutual aid is about constructing positive rather than "spoiled" social identities, constructing a "normative narrative community" (Rappaport 1993), and embarking on a "recovery journey" in which a person holistically lives life through his "problem." David Robinson and Stuart Henry said it best in 1977:

> In self-help groups, the problem is not separated off from everyday
> activities by buildings or chemicals. The treaters are not separated off
> by education, class or expertise. Nothing is hived-off, boxed away or
> cut out. In self-help helping the problem is *integrated* with life; the

treated is the treater and the treatment is to find a new way of living, incorporating the problem into one's everyday experience. This is done by providing a continuous form of care and concern through a network of friendship that itself permeates everyday living and closes the distance between normal everyday living and having problems. Thus, rather than *living* everyday life and *having* problems, self-help group members live their everyday life *through* their problems. All the changes in perception about the severity of problems, the availability of help, the significance of asking for help, of not discontinuing help, require people to change their everyday lives. This is what we mean when we say self-help groups transform people. (1977, 121)

Transforming people by changing their everyday lives also includes the commons, creating a normalizing community in which people with a stigma can see themselves as whole persons who have a flaw or limitation. In the commons people can explore their humanness, develop intimacy with experiential peers, undertake a journey of recovery that can encompass the spiritual, develop organizational skills to participate in civil society, participate in an identity-oriented (new) social movement, and contribute to their community's store of social capital.

In the 1990s professional observers have recognized the differences in paradigms between self-help/mutual aid and professional services, but the metaparadigm just described is not well established. The possibilities for relationships between self-help/mutual aid and the professionally based health and human services system is now couched in terms of the inherent tensions between them because of the different value premises, assumptions, ethos, nature of the helping relationship, and structure of relationships.[17]

Even such a seemingly simple matter as emotional expressivity is so different between self-helpers and professionals that chasms develop in attempts to communicate. An interesting report chronicles the well-meaning government-employed professionals who tried to implement participation in policymaking for consumers of mental health services. The intensity of emotional expression among the wounded consumer/survivors contrasted so sharply with professional reserve that the professionals often perceived the consumer/survivors as having "bad manners." The outside sociological observer chronicled the problematic communication that developed, showing that emotional expressiveness is far from bad manners (Church 1996).

Self-help groups, especially those for medical conditions and rare diseases (excluding 12-step groups), often have the latest information about diagnostic tests, treatments, and other aspects of their condition. The average practitioner is unlikely to be up-to-date on many of these infrequently occurring conditions. For example, Temple Grandin (1995) tells her story of recovering from autism and suggests to readers that the self-help group—the Autism Society of America—is likely to have the latest information.

Self-helpers' complaints about professionals lie in part with professionals who claim specialized knowledge they do not have. Marsha Schubert, a special education teacher, helped parents of intellectually gifted children with learning disabilities to start a self-help group. Several years later she enlisted the leaders to collaborate on research about what experiential knowledge the parents had gained through their participation. The parent co-researchers were responsible for the most striking finding: parents differentiated between generalist professionals who had no specific knowledge of learning disabilities of gifted students and specialist professionals who had such expert knowledge. Parents readily used the experts but avoided the generalists (see Schubert and Borkman 1994). Other incidents are reported of people with rare diseases banding together in computer-based chat groups on the Internet to obtain the latest information and to direct their treatment; they know more than generalist professionals (see Franklin 1998).

Despite or because of the inherent tensions arising from different paradigms and worldviews, the relationships between self-helpers and their commons on the one side and professionals and agencies on the other represent challenges that can be tackled: some will be fruitful, others frustrating or unsettling. There is much to be learned on both or all sides. Especially important and neglected is learning how self-help/mutual aid can inform and enlighten professional practices; the self-helpers have experiential expertise about living with their condition and are smart consumers about receiving professional services. Professionals and agencies can benefit from the experientially informed self-helpers who critique formal services and suggest improvements.

Chapter 5

The Evolution of a Group for People Who Stutter

W<small>E KNOW LITTLE</small> about how self-help groups develop or what organizational life cycles they follow. Established and viable mutual help groups possess a meaning perspective or framework that they have tested and used over time. Fledgling groups have to create a meaning perspective about their problem or borrow and adapt one from another group. A group that does not have a meaning perspective that is satisfactory to its members is unlikely to survive.

The story is told here of how the first viable mutual help group for people who stutter (PWS) in the United States began and evolved over a seventeen-year period. The story is constructed from four research studies of the group conducted between 1966 and 1983.[1] Instead of presenting findings as an analytical case study, this is an experiment in constructing a narrative about the evolution of a group.[2]

I use the narrative technique because self-help groups tell stories as a major means of conveying information and understanding (as described in Rappaport 1993, chaps. 1 and 2; Kennedy and Humphreys 1994; Humphreys and Rappaport 1994). Compared with conventional, linear third-person social science reporting, the narrative form conveys to the reader the emotional impact of a story. The narrative form enables the reader to better understand how meaning perspectives develop: both the group's meaning perspective and my own framework applied to understanding theirs.

The narrative is based on actual persons who were leaders and members of the group, although pseudonyms have been assigned to preserve confidentiality. The real names of two professionals, Joseph Sheehan and Charles Van

Riper, now deceased, are retained as are the actual names of the Edinburgh Masker and the Hollins College fluency shaping program.[3]

The story of each period in the group's evolution shows some of the complexity and the wide range of issues dealt with in the group at any point in time. (See Denzin and Lincoln [1994] for a discussion of the uses of narratives in social science research.) Not all the complexity of the group's development can be portrayed in a short narrative, of course, but an effort has been made to cover enough issues to give a sense of them all; these include ideas about the meaning perspective—how the problem is defined, its resolution, and members' identity as well as the composition and functioning of the group. The story shows the kinds of issues that dominate during each time period. It is necessarily selective and compressed.

Implicit in this narrative is a developmental view, examining how the group evolves its meaning perspective and associated experiential knowledge as well as its organizational structure; these issues will be analyzed in chapter 6. As you read the story, keep in mind the four aspects of the meaning perspective:

1. How do we (the group) define the nature of our problem of stuttering? For example, is it physical, psychological or learned? Is it curable or incurable?
2. What is a satisfactory way of resolving our stuttering problem? For example, what are available therapies, treatments, or means to solve or resolve the stuttering problem? How well do they work?
3. What are our characteristics as people who stutter—how does our personal identity relate to our problem of stuttering? What social identity is allotted to us by society?
4. What social technology should we use to facilitate our problem solving?

In addition, the narrative covers such organizational issues as:

1. Governance and organizational structure: who with what authority controls the group and sets the operating rules? Is the group member-led, professionally controlled, or a hybrid? How much dependence does the group have on external sources? (These issues are described in chapter 4.)
2. What is the role of a human service agency or a professional, if any, in developing and controlling the group (also described in chapter 4)?
3. Who is responsible for leading meetings and doing other tasks necessary to maintain the organization? Are members experienced and willing to assume leadership positions to maintain the organization? How are

potential members enticed to participate and contribute to organizational maintenance in this voluntary setting? Who and how many
members develop skills associated with maintaining a self-help/mutual
aid commons? (See table 3.1.)

4. External goals and values: self-help groups are membership associations,
   oriented to directly benefiting their members. Do they also evolve
   external goals to help others or remain inwardly focused? If external
   goals are developed, are they for education of the public or professionals,
   personal advocacy, or social advocacy?

5. To what extent does support develop outside the meetings with a
   community of friendships? Friendships are an important part of the
   social bonds that entice members to participate and contribute to the
   group. What kinds of friendships and informal relationships are encouraged through social activities and the like?

The story begins in 1966, when the group was founded by a fluent speech
therapist and two of his clients in stuttering therapy. It is presented as snap-
shots of the group over six time periods: 1966, 1967, 1969, 1971, 1976, and
1983. The first view is of an initial meeting of the group in 1966; another
meeting is described nine months later in 1967. The second part of the story
depicts the group in 1969 and 1971, when it is stable, developed, and effective in helping members; the third part of the story occurs in 1976, when the
group, now ten years old and still effective for its members, has broadened to
initiate a national coalition of groups like itself; the fourth and final meeting
takes place in 1983, when the group is seventeen years old and disintegrating. The legacy of this once-thriving group lives on, however, in the national
organization that was developed in the mid-1970s and its offshoots. This pioneering effort also sparked connections that resulted in other self-help/mu-
tual aid groups for people who stutter.

An East Coast Group Searches for a Perspective on Stuttering, 1966

*A meeting of the newly formed group in 1966 is described. The fledgling group is
developing its goals, values, activities, and meaning perspective. Within this first year
the group decides on a governance structure, adopts some external goals, and its
basic social technology (supportive safe meetings in which people can talk and stutter without being judged). The nonstuttering speech therapist sponsor of the group
hosts meetings at the university clinic where he is a professor. He is an open-minded
professional who is willing to help the group get started, but he wants them to be-*

come autonomous. The professional sponsor warns the group against being friends or having social events outside the context of the group.

AN INITIAL MEETING OF THE GROUP, 1966

In a speech and hearing clinic in a metropolitan university on the East Coast, a group of ten people who stutter are meeting; also included is their sponsor John, a fluent speech therapist who conducts stuttering therapy at the clinic. The cofounders, Mick and Dick (both of whom stutter), had met in John's waiting room between therapy appointments where they had come up with the idea for the group. John is sympathetic to the idea of stutterers' meeting together and agrees to help them organize as long as they do not become too dependent on him. John is also concerned that these stutterers not get too involved socially with one another, lest they end up as a "huddle-together" group that Dr. Joseph Sheehan, a renowned psychologist and ex-stutterer, has warned against. John has talked to Dr. Sheehan; he had started a group for his clinic patients in the early 1950s, but the group deteriorated into a self-pitying retreat from the fluent world and he stopped referring clients to it.

The first meeting. John, who separately is giving stuttering therapy to almost everyone present, makes a few introductory remarks about the possibilities of the group and his willingness to sponsor it if the group strives to develop the skills to become autonomous. Mick and Dick are especially excited by the warm compassionate attitude that John has helped establish during this meeting. Dick, who only knows a few of the people present, thinks to himself: I instantly feel comfortable with these people!

The chair opens up tonight's topic—"Why are you here? What do you want to get from these meetings?" Sally, one of the few women, says that coming to this group is the first time she has ever talked to another stutterer. She feels relieved to see so many normal-looking and accomplished people, to find out that "we are-are not black sh-sheep or oddballs or anything." Dick stutters slightly but comfortably as he says, "Just giving me social interaction. Giving me the opportunity of feeling like a human being!" Maggie and Jonah, new to stuttering therapy and to hearing a fellow stutterer, are impressed with Dick. They hope to be able to talk as fearlessly as he does someday.

Ned chimes in, "I myself am not a stutterer. I have a fourteen-year-old son who is. I joined the group with the two-fold objective of better informing myself to help him and of becoming useful in combating the general problem."

As they go systematically around the circle, two young men in their twenties are silently shaking their head that they do not want to say anything. One looks frightened. Others respond empathetically, having felt frightened themselves when they first heard someone else stutter severely.

A few people do not sound disfluent, an unknowledgable person would wonder if they were people who stutter. Other people stumble over a few words only, but their disfluency does not impede their flow of talking. A few, including informed leaders, have marked disfluency. They are extremely slow to articulate a whole sentence. While some are a little disquieted by the severe stuttering, a general air of tolerance and kindness in the room continues to support those participants with disfluencies. People are given all the time they need to complete their verbalization—an important principle that was immediately established and ensures a safe space for building an effective dialogue for people with stuttering problems.

Conflict immediately emerges over how often they should meet—Mick and Dick want informal weekly meetings so people have a chance to talk with one another about their experiences with stuttering and get support. Others feel that a monthly educational meeting is adequate. Behind the conflict over times to meet is the important issue of whether or not this will be a support group of people sharing their experiences or an educational session with experts telling them about therapies. The idea of a circle of sharing and support wins out, and the new group begins meeting weekly.

A 1967 Meeting: Organizational Problems and Issues about Therapy

Nine months later the meetings are well established. Participants vary extensively in the frequency and other patterns of attendance. Although the group has already achieved status as a nonprofit organization and has elected officers, issues of inadequate leadership are surfacing.

In the late 1960s and continuing through today, many theories of the cause of stuttering are available but unproved. Similarly, many kinds of speech therapy for stuttering are available, but all seem to provide only temporary relief from stuttering. Moreover, many unproven commercial gimmicks are advertised by quacks. The legitimate and concerned speech therapist sponsor of the group teaches the "nonavoidance approach" to stuttering, developed by speech therapists who stutter, to the group, but participants differ in how acceptable they find it. The "nonavoidance approach" is difficult to translate into concrete activities.

NINE MONTHS LATER IN 1967

In a weekly meeting in early October, twenty-six attendees sit in a circle. Mick, the chair of the meeting, announces that after the informal sharing time, the second half of the meeting will be a business meeting. He asks if all dues-paying members got their newsletter in the mail and if they saw the article on the soul of a stutterer by Stan. He also announces that plans for a television show featuring their group are completed. Dick's father, who works at a television station, has gotten the group an invitation to put on a public service program about the problem of stuttering. The script has been written by John and four other members (three of whom are officers) and the taping is next week.

The leader announces that two weeks from tonight they will have Sam Jones, director of a speech therapy clinic at a local university, as the guest speaker. Members are urged to attend and ask questions of Jones during the question and answer period.

Mick describes the topic of tonight's meeting: Have you had speech therapy? What kind of therapy was it and how helpful was it? Sally starts the circle of sharing. She has had two different kinds of speech therapy, one in grade school, and one in college. Now she is pursuing stuttering therapy with John, the group's sponsor. She recounts that the first therapy she had didn't really seem like therapy—it was reading from a book mostly. While in college she went to a speech clinic; she learned to speak fluently in the therapist's office but began stuttering when she went to the grocery store. Sally thought something was wrong with her because she stuttered in the store.

Jonah, a college student and next in turn, has never had any therapy and admits he is afraid to go. Stan, a twenty-five-year-old bookkeeper, talks about the three previous forms of speech therapy he has had; like Sally, he could be fluent in the therapist's office but not at work or on the street. One therapy, based on a principle of distraction, left him stutter-free; for six months he was blissful to be so fluent but then his stuttering returned to its previous level. John, the speech therapist, acknowledged that Stan's experience was all too common. Others around the room share similar stories of several kinds of speech therapy that worked for a while, then the gains disappeared. The participants commonly thought something was wrong with them when the fluency gained in therapy did not work in everyday life or the gains disappeared after a few months. About half the participants had had some form of speech therapy, often two or more types, and a few had had psychotherapy or hypnosis.

"What is this nonavoidance approach I keep hearing about?" asks a relatively new member named Harry. John explains that their consistently disappointing experiences with many stuttering therapies are typical. The vain search for fluency is a dead end. He believes the nonavoidance approach to stuttering is the most viable. No cure is known, but the nonavoidance philosophy is learning to accept that you have a stuttering problem rather than avoiding it. Then, you can focus your energies on learning to talk, reduce your fear of talking, and learn to stutter comfortably. Many people find their disfluency is paradoxically diminished in the process. John explains that he follows the nonavoidance philosophy of stuttering in his therapy, which is based on the writings of Dr. Joseph Sheehan and Dr. Charles Van Riper;[4] he has studied with Van Riper and knows both of them as outstanding pioneers in developing the nonavoidance philosophy. Both Joseph Sheehan and Charles Van Riper are recovered stutterers. John's speech therapy helps ease blocks, gives a better air flow, and helps a person stutter more easily; it is not a panacea or a cure. During the second half of the gathering, Ralph, a fifty-year-old married lawyer, leads the business meeting. He announces that the group's application to be legally incorporated as a nonprofit organization has been accepted and the name Caring Group on Stuttering is now legal. However, an organizational crisis has developed. Although seven people were elected as officers barely six months ago, they have been inactive and have been asked to resign. They have done so. We need people who are willing to be active leaders, he says. We need nominations for new officers in order to hold an election. He continues: I know many of you have never held an office; you have let your stuttering keep you from participating. But we need your help; you can learn as you go and John, our special therapist friend, is willing to teach us how to run the organization.

Mick and Stan, previously on the board, volunteer to run for reelection as does John, the speech therapist who had been one of three vice presidents. Newcomers Jonah and Harry offer to be nominated, and with some coaxing, the slate is filled. John ends the meeting by saying that despite this setback in leadership, he is enthusiastic about the group's potential, including the members' capacity to run their own organization by themselves one day. He compliments the group on its efforts.

After the meeting Jonah and Harry talk to Stan about what is involved in being an officer, since they have never been one. Conversation drifts to embarrassing moments they had stuttering the previous week. They turn out the lights and lock up as the last ones to leave.

Developing Collective Experiences

Two years later, the Caring Group is well established and running smoothly. Seasoned members have learned the value to themselves of presenting educational programs to the public; the leaders and other active members grow and change more than the inactive or irregular attenders. They explore new identities as people who stutter. The long-term members have become confident of what they know from personal experience about stuttering as they have developed their collective experience.

Governance is clearly in the hands of people who stutter. A new Advisory and Honorary Board has been created for professional friends.

A MEETING IN EARLY 1969

Early arrivals chat as old friends before the meeting starts. For example, Betty introduces the newcomer Ronald, a thirty-year-old, to her friend Ellen, who has attended for two years and is a forty-year-old mother of two children. Ronald asks Ellen, "How did you react when you first came here?" Ellen replied with enthusiasm, "It is/was love at first sight. Because people lis-listened to me and they didn't cor-correct my-my speech. I-I was listened to, I w-was left alone to say whatever I-I wanted to to say and it was taken seriously!" Ronald and Betty share how they reacted—Ronald is upset to hear people who stutter severely whereas Betty is positive, similar to Ellen.

The meeting begins with seventeen people sitting in a circle. The success of last week's public meeting for parents of young stutterers and other interested people is applauded. Dick, cofounder and past president, was master of ceremonies at the public meeting and said that thirty people had attended, mostly parents of children who stuttered. Four long-term members, Stan, Harry, Mick, and Sally had spoken as well as John, their speech therapist adviser. The ten-minute film about stuttering problems of children that had been shown was well received. Ronald was amazed to hear how his four peers had so casually spoken in public. He knew he could never do that—or could he? If they could, maybe he could get over his fear someday.

The leader, Harry, then began the main portion of the meeting by announcing that the topic for discussion was going to be difficulties talking on the telephone. Sam feels a little impatient, since he remembers that telephone troubles is a topic they discussed about eight months ago, and he would like more variety. But, continues Harry, Ralph and Stan asked to have a discussion on self-concept and identity as a stutterer.

Stan, a seasoned member, begins by saying, "I u-used to think there was something seriously wrong with me, but when I met other stutterers and found they were so nice and came in so many different personality types, I could no longer believe stuttering was anything to be ashamed of as such."

Joan, next in the circle, says, "It is exciting for me to know I am not alone. I am n-not weird. So many of you I like and admire are also stutterers and that means I can like and admire myself."

When it is his turn, Tom, a middle-aged man who began attending six months ago, expresses himself very fluently.

> I faced my speech problem ten years ago for the first time and my
> reward was a degree of comfort in speech. I was drawn to the group,

not because I could not communicate comfortably, but because I felt like a stutterer still, even though I did not sound like one. I am learning from this group that while I was not running away from the problem of stuttering, I was running away from everything else. I think I have stopped running away. I am taking tennis lessons and seriously dating for the first time in my life.

Then the newcomer Willy expresses his feelings in hesitant slow speech, punctuated by disfluencies.

I-I have enough insecurity and inferiority feelings for an army; I su-su-suppose we all do. Most pppeople learn to liv-live with them. As I walk through life feeling the lowest of the llllow, I wonder how much, consciously or subconsciously, I am blaming my stuttering for my inferiority, h-h-how much I need my stuttering to hang all my other f-f-f-faults on.

Others nod their heads in empathy.
Ellen speaks passionately during her turn.

Some people expect the group to benefit them but they aren't willing to meet the group halfway, and try to help themselves. Some seem to think the group can wave a magic wand over them, and transform them overnight into a self-confident, nonstuttering person. This simply cannot be done. If the person who stutters wants help, she must first decide she is going to do all she can to help herself; otherwise, she is defeated before she has really begun. I did not change until I was willing to help myself and stop blaming my stuttering and everything else. Now I can ask you for help.

Judd, a twenty-year-old who has had speech therapy at a local military clinic, says, "I came to the Caring Group for a year before I offered to help out in any way. I sat and said very little. I was really scared. Now that I am volunteering to help and taking some risks with speaking, I feel better about myself. I find it very slow and painful to change, though."

Harry, an officer and a seasoned member, comments, "I think stuttering dominates our life; we are full of self-pity and feel like the 'walking wounded.' All we think about is our guilt, shame, and embarrassment about stuttering. We don't live life but are consumed by preoccupation with stuttering or avoiding our blocks and moments of stuttering. I am less preoccupied with stuttering after several years in the Caring Group, and I find being active and helping others gets me outside myself."

Mick then stuttered comfortably about how he had accepted that he stuttered and did not try to avoid stuttering as he had before. The newcomer

Charles asks, "I get the idea you don't think a cure is possible? If you are accepting that you stutter, why are we here?" The secretary responds that "our activities are designed to personally involve each person with a commitment to himself and a commitment to face up to his stuttering. A lot of us who have been with the group for years doubt that searching for a cure is a useful way to spend our energies. We are better off facing our stuttering and not letting it interfere with our lives so much."

The group usually has a two- to three-month plan of topics, related to upsetting and painful aspects of living with stuttering such as talking on the telephone, talking in public, the listener's reaction to stuttering, issues in talking to families about stuttering, or sex and the single stutterer. Some meetings review and critique various speech therapies, or mechanical devices to avoid stuttering or other sure-fire commercial gimmicks. Parties and other social events are held once or twice a year, but some people are ambivalent about them because of what they have heard about Dr. Sheehan's admonition that support groups for stutterers will become retreats from living if members become too friendly with one another.

The speech therapist adviser, John, announces that he has confirmed that thirty-three professionals will be advisory and honorary members to the Caring Group. These professionals, John adds, mainly speech pathologist clinicians but some researchers and psychologists, will help legitimate the Caring Group and will "look good" on the stationery letterhead. They won't have any say in how the group is run—that is for the members—and most of them will never even attend a meeting.

At the end of the meeting they go around in turn saying their full names—a slow and tortuous process for many. Nick hates saying his name, but it is part of his identity. Practicing a difficult speaking task in this safe nonjudgmental environment will benefit him in the long run, he muses.

After the meeting, friends chat about their week's activities and some welcome newcomers, drawing them out to get acquainted.

A Fully Developed Meaning Perspective

The group is now five years old, well organized, and effective in helping involved participants. Differences between newcomers and seasoned members, especially leaders, are striking. Seasoned members trust their experiential knowledge of stuttering, and they are confident enough to critically question the value of specific stuttering therapies and commercial gimmicks. Newcomers often believe that a cure (that is, fluency) is possible, while the veterans who have tried many alternatives are more accepting of the "nonavoidance approach" to stuttering. Participants hold differing opinions about fluency, the value of stuttering therapy, the acceptability of the "nonavoidance approach," and so forth; the group respects diversity of opinion. Some members are friends, and social events are held. Some do not understand the importance of having meetings to attend to the group's organizational maintenance. Governance is more solidly controlled by members, and the nonstuttering professionals like the speech therapist sponsor are not allowed to be officers.

A MEETING IN 1971

John, the group's adviser, shows up for the first time in weeks. He is warmly greeted by many participants; they are obviously fond of him and appreciate his compassion in helping them with their stuttering problem. John announces that he has been getting letters from people around the country who want to start or have tried to start groups like the Caring Group; a list of them is in the last newsletter. They ask for help and inspiration in getting a group going. He would appreciate hearing from anyone who wants to help him answer the letters and send out materials. He tells about a group in North Carolina that has been meeting for several months, trying out the format and topics of the Caring Group. Several members who are from the military clinic offer to help.

The meeting begins with the president making an announcement that they will have a speaker from Dale Carnegie next week. He continues by saying that the night's topic is "stuttering therapy: is it for you?" Ralph, the secretary, will start with a review of a new book written by a professional speech therapist about another kind of stuttering therapy. Ralph proceeds to describe the therapy and how it is conducted, concluding with his own opinion that it is another therapy that is unlikely to work in everyday life. Joe, the vice president, then agrees that from what Ralph has said, it's another version of distraction therapy that won't work in the long run.

Stan then reads from a letter that Harold Berger is distributing the Edinburgh Masker from his foundation in the Midwest and recalls that Berger was at the group's national convention last year to demonstrate it. "What is it?" Harold asks. Phyllis explains that it is a tiny device put in the ear that masks one's speaking so the stutterer's delayed auditory feedback problem is avoided. "Does it work or is it more quack stuff?" Harold wants to know. Phyllis believes that "it is on the up and up and I know a couple of people who use it. But it produces speech with an unnatural cadence. I sure would not use it!"

Some newcomers like Gil and Marie voice concern about the negative review given this speech therapy, the Edinburgh Masker, and by implication other stuttering therapies. Veteran group members reassure them, saying that all members should try the stuttering therapies they are interested in and sat-isfy themselves whether they work or not—the group is certainly not trying to discourage anyone from seeking stuttering therapy. And the long-term mem-bers also point out that other kinds of therapy, like psychotherapy, can be con-sidered. Joe, as a matter of fact, is one of the few members who is in psychotherapy. Some techniques, such as hypnosis, they do not recommend.

The conversation turns to the issue of whether the search for fluency is a fruitful one. The president and another old-timer in the group say the issue is not fluency, but learning to accept that one has a permanent stuttering prob-lem. In fact, the more you search for fluency, the less you may gain it. Some seasoned group members nod in agreement, reflecting that it took them sev-eral years to accept the seemingly paradoxical approach to stuttering. Other more recent attendees disagree with this approach and think that the atti-tude that stuttering is permanent is fatalistic. They argue that one will stop trying if that attitude is adopted. Just because one or two dozen stuttering thera-pies have not worked does not mean that none will work. Fluency is the im-portant goal for which to strive. There is a wide variety of opinions about the attainability of fluency. For some newcomers the idea that their stuttering may be incurable is demoralizing and unacceptable. But the seasoned members of the group recount their experiences and those of other members who have tried three or five or even seven stuttering therapies with dismal results. The seasoned members feel that they are personally not demoralized because they no longer search for a cure. In fact, they are energized because they have a constructive way of approaching their stuttering: they are gaining self-respect and confidence by being in the Caring Group; they are getting involved in the regular world; stuttering is diminishing its hold on their lives; they are less fearful of talking to fluent speakers; and they love the friendships and ca-maraderie of the Caring Group. Through the heated discussion, respect for others' opinions is maintained. Before the meeting ends, the president an-nounces that the by-law changes have been approved by ballot: only a per-son who stutters can be an officer (implying that the speech therapist adviser can no longer hold office). John smiles, saying that the group is really becoming independent, which he thinks is great.

Marie, a twenty-year-old college student who is a client in John's stutter-ing therapy, asks why the group had a business meeting last week; she feels it takes time away from working on their stuttering. The secretary, Ralph, pa-tiently explains that the group has to take care of its organizational needs or it could dissolve. Ellen agrees with Marie that maybe too much time is spent on organizational issues, which can be boring. Ralph fills in some history of the group for Marie. Four years ago they spent half or more of their time on developing a constitution and bylaws and other aspects of the nonprofit organization for almost a year. This time commitment was necessary to get the group properly functioning. Ellen disagrees, saying that she remembers the group faltered because members started dropping out during this time. Newcomers would not return after one or two visits. As far as she was concerned, too much time was spent on the dry details of organization.

The meeting ends with the regular custom of everyone saying his or her full name out loud. As usual, friends chat after the meeting about the gains they have made and the risks they are taking in their jobs, leisure-time activities, or family.

An Autonomous Mature Open Learning Group

The group is now ten years old, effective in helping some involved participants, especially leaders, change their stuttering behavior and self-identity. Members view themselves as normal people who have a minor defect, stuttering; this defect does not rule their life. The group has broadened its goals to include advocacy. It has helped in the formation of a national organization for groups patterned after itself; the groups maintain their local autonomy. A new form of stuttering therapy has been located that promises fluency, but at the cost of an unnatural monotone speech; members have sharply different reactions to it.

A MEETING IN 1976

Five years later at the same clinic, five friends greet one another warmly before the meeting starts. Dick, a cofounder who has not been to a meeting in several months, is hugged by Ellen and enthusiastically greeted by Joe, who also has not been to a meeting for months. Carol, the current president, asks, "How was your trip to Japan?" "Great," answers Dick, "you'll hear all about it in my re-report tonight—I'll also t-t-talk about the national convention of the National Caring Group in Illinois last m-m-m-month. I enjoyed rooming with you, Joe, at the convention. Incidentally, Ellen is doing a great job editing the National Caring Group's news-news-newsletter." Ellen lights up with a smile. The conversation continues as others join them before the meeting.

Larry, a forty-year-old veterinarian and infrequent attender, arrives and hesitantly joins in. Relative newcomers Shari, a twenty-year-old secretary who has attended the past eight months, and Harold, a twenty-five-year-old auto mechanic who has been only four or five times before, arrive right before the meeting starts. Carol starts the meeting after the twelve people are settled comfortably in the usual circle. She welcomes special guests, saying that "Dick, a cofounder and past president who is now an officer of the National Caring

Group (and our delegate to the National Group), is someone we don't see much anymore. Joe is also one of our past presidents who was very active in developing the Caring Group during its early y-years whom we also don't see often any more." She announces the topics for the meetings for next month, including "What Are Our Avoidance Patterns?," "Stuttering and Self-Assertion," "Stuttering and Friendships," and "Personal Goals—What do we want and what are we doing to achieve them?"

A final announcement concerns the current campaigns to inform parents of children who stutter about the disorder and to reach local speech therapists to inform them about the group. Ellen reports that the project to send packets of written material to parents who write for them is going satisfactorily. In contrast, the response to the one hundred letters written to local speech therapists offering to inform them about the Caring Group and how it will work with them and their clients has been disappointing—no responses have been received after one month.

Carol suggests that they begin with a period to let people share where they are before the special program tonight on the self-help group in Japan. As they share in turn, the participants express where they are personally. Joe says,

> After eight years in the Caring Group and psychotherapy, and all, I-I-I am aware of the lit-little blocks that I still have. I'm aware that they pass, that they are not the most important thing to happen to me. I'm aware of things to do to relax myself before sp-sp-speaking in a situation. . . . I have a new philosophy about dealing with my stuttering. When I'm beginning a new relationship with someone, to very shortly, not right off the bat, talk about st-stuttering and mention the fact that I do st-stutter, and get that out in the open.

Carol, Harold, and Shari smile and make eye contact with each other. They are thinking the same thing—they are so impressed with Joe! How courageous he is! How self-confident! How comfortable with his disfluencies!

Dick talks about the part he is rehearsing in a play in a community theater. How exciting it is to participate with fluent people as a regular person. "I am living life now," he says, "instead of thinking about how fluent or not I am. I used to be so passive—blaming my troubles on my stuttering—I was too scared and had no self-confidence to try out for a play. But a lot of us are passive when we first come here."

Ellen slowly and disfluently says, "I-I know-know I have the r-r-r-right to speak in p-p-public—to take as much t-t-t-time as I need in p-p-p-public—for example, in a cafeteria line to express what I need and not hhhhhhurry up ending ending ending up getting something I don't want. The Caring Group taught me t-t-t-that." The veteran members nod their heads in agreement. Carol says excitedly, "I am going to the stuttering therapy at Hollins College this summer. Its precision shaping fluency program. I met several people with stuttering problems at the last conference who talk fluently after taking that therapy." Joe asks her: "But don't Hollins College graduates have to work hard to keep their fluency? Don't they have to continue to do exercises or they lose their fluency? Don't they talk in a monotone—no emotional expressiveness or you revert to your disfluencies?" Carol reluctantly agrees, saying, "I'd rather be fluent and talk in a monotone than be expressive and stutter."

Dick then enthusiastically reports on his trip to Japan to attend a conference of the members of a self-help group like the Caring Group—also described in the newsletter of the National Caring Group. In addition, he reports on the national convention in the Midwest. "We now have eight groups that are part of the National Caring Group on Stuttering—groups in such places as Baltimore, Florida, Michigan, and Illinois." Joe and Carol are very excited to add their perspectives on the convention and the other wonderful people they met from around the country. So many inspiring activities and success stories!

As the meeting ends, Carol announces the details of the October retreat at a farm and reminds them to bring their families or friends to the Christmas party. She reminds people they are all invited for coffee right after the meeting at the regular coffee shop. They close in the usual manner, each in turn saying his or her name out loud. The few who linger to chat aren't going out with the others; the rest leave for coffee.

AT COFFEE AFTER THE MEETING

At the coffee shop, Carol, Joe, Dick, and Shari take a table for four. Larry and Ellen arrive later, sitting within hearing distance at a table for two. At the larger table, Joe asks Dick and Carol if they have been in contact with Ralph, an early leader who stopped attending several years before. Dick responds that he has heard that Ralph is very busy volunteering with a legal aid group to do trial work—"you know his specialty is patent law, which puts him behind a desk with lots of papers, seldom talking to anyone. Now he is excited about developing as a trial lawyer. Did you know he joined Toastmasters, the group where people give speeches all the time? Do you remember Ralph brought Toastmasters up a number of times at the group as something we should look into—but we never did."

As Joe and Dick talk about the early days of the Caring Group, Shari hesitantly asks Carol, "Should I go to st-stuttering ther-therapy? You know the ffffarming area I came from in W-W-West Virginia had no therapy for stutterers. So I have never had it. Some people really bad-mouth it. What-What do you think I-I should do?" Carol responds, "I think you could see a speech th-therapist if you think it's right for you. But-But I can't tell you which one to go to; you have to decide—ttttalk to people about their experiences, read about therapies, find out about rates of success, and so on. Then-then decide."

At the small table, Larry is complaining in low whispers to Ellen so he will not be overheard.

> I only came to meetings per-periodically because I-I-I had a disagree-ment with Dick and felt angry about that. This was several years ago. He-He manipulated behind the scenes so I didn't get an officer's position. I also wanted some new ideas brought into the group, but the leaders didn't really listen to me. I wanted a psychiatrist to come talk to the ggggroup to get another viewpoint and brought it up a couple of times but-but never pressed it. At another time I-I was head of a committee looking into hypnotism—in 1971 or 1972 a hypnotist came here wanting to-to work up some program but it never got too far. Guess I'm-I'm still a little angry.

Ellen is sympathetic, but she explains that her experience with the Caring Group has been different. She feels that she has gotten a great deal from the Caring Group—it has changed her life. She confides, "YYYou know the religious cccconcept of grace, which is something you can-cannot earn but a gift that is given to-to you. I-I-I-I got the gift of grace from the Caring Group—the love, the magic, the sp-sp-spirit of the Caring Group that-that-that trans-forms people. Of course, I-I wouldn't use that term-terminology around lots of the members—they will have nothing to do with anything that sounds like r-r-religion or the sp-sp-spiritual."

After their coffee, they all part with good-natured humor and expressions of fellowship.

Caring Group Diminution: Failure or Community Resource?

Seventeen years after its initiation, the group is disintegrating. Only four people attend an infrequent meeting. The group split in half when some members left to form a "therapy maintenance group." The speech therapist adviser no longer refers potential members, because he has left the university. The few remaining members lack leadership or energy to recruit new members and revitalize the group, or the national-level organization absorbs their energy. The national organization has be-come assertive as an advocate for people who stutter. Two other national organiza-tions have developed, a membership organization on the West Coast and a federation of groups on the East Coast.

AN INFREQUENT MEETING IN 1983

It is 7:30 P.M. on Wednesday at the center. Only Maura and Phillip are there in time for the meeting. Lou shows up at 7:35; Ellen apologetically comes in at 7:45.

Maura opens the meeting of four people at 7:50. She is filling in for the president, Vicki, who is out of town. There is no planned topic for tonight. "What would people like to talk about? What is bothering them?" she asks. Phillip speaks up—"I am interested in what is going on with the-the Caring Group and the National Group. I moved to the West Coast four y-y-years ago and have not sub-subscribed to the National Caring Group Newsletter. This is my first time b-b-back. What's been happening? I joined the American Stuttering Program on the West Coast and have been going to meetings there— it's different than the Caring Group."

Ellen shows them the latest newsletter for the National Caring Group on Stuttering which she just finished editing—it is in the mail to subscribers now. Maura suggests maybe they could go through some of the highlights of the newsletter to become more current. Is that okay with everyone? Phillip is excited by it. Lou smiles and offers to read parts of the newsletter—he mentions that he does not stutter badly when he reads even though many do. But he stutters when he sings, unlike many other people who stutter. He's used to being different, even from other people who stutter, he jokes.

Maura suggests they go around and introduce themselves since most of them do not seem to know one another. She begins, saying that she has been coming to the group for three years but does not come often since she started college at night last fall. The group gave her enough confidence to go to college, she adds.

Phillip says that the only person at the meeting that he knows is Ellen, who has been in the group almost from the beginning; he has always respected Ellen for her wonderful articles and editing of the newsletter and for her courage in facing her stuttering problems. Ellen smiles appreciatively at the compliment and says she has been coming since the group was three years old. Phillip explains that he had been the secretary of the group five years ago, before he moved to the West Coast. Lou says he has been coming on and off for two years.

Lou looks at the newsletter: "Dick—isn't he one of our cofounders?— stepped down from his position as secretary of the national. He has an article— looks really interesting—on stuttering as involving four aspects. I'll read what he says." He reads,

> Stuttering, we've all heard, is not a speech disorder; it's a communication disorder. Communication consists of four broad areas: speech,

nonverbal communication, self-concept (the feelings about self that the speaker presents to the listener), and interpersonal contact (the degree to which the speaker feels in contact with the listener). It is widely known that in a stuttered block, there are breakdowns in *all four* of these communication areas. In a stuttered block: a person's gesture ceases, a person's self-concept lowers as he or she feels guilt or anger with themselves; contact with the other ceases as all energy is brought inside the self to force one's way through the block. It is also well known that breakdowns in any of the other communication areas seem to cause breakdowns in speech. Stutterers universally report that they stutter more when they sense a loss of the listener or when they do not feel good about themselves. The four areas of communication seem inextricably tied together. And a therapy that works on only one of the four areas seems doomed to failure.

Lou continues summarizing announcements from the newsletter. "Dr. Gerald Diego, an industrial psychologist, writes a long letter about losing his job as a counselor in a middle school because of his stuttering. He fought it with the State Human Relations Commission, but after two years they dismissed his case for lack of evidence. Gerald Diego's stuttering increased when he felt so bad about himself; a vicious circle, he calls it."

The announcements continue. "The national officers spoke about what kind of research needs to be done by the National Institute of Neurological and Communication Disorders and Stroke, National Institutes of Health (NIH). They were invited with twenty other voluntary groups—hearing impaired, cleft palates, deaf, laryngectomies, and so on—to a two-day conference at NIH. Our officers criticized stuttering research for only covering the speech aspect of the communication process and leaving out the other three areas—self-concept, nonspeech communicative behavior, and self-other interaction." "Exciting," interjects Maura.

"Sad news to read that Dr. Joseph Sheehan died." Maura comments, "He spoke at the last convention of the National Caring Group on Stuttering. Wasn't he a major professional figure that developed the nonavoidance philosophy?" Ellen answered, "Yes, and-and he was very respected be-be-because he also had stutt-stuttered so he really knew-knew what he-he was t-t-talking about. But-But he also misled us. T-t-t-telling self-help groups n-n-not to be sociable, or have parties. We should not become fr-friends with each other and-and go out for c-c-coffee after meetings. He was sure wr-wrong about that."

Phillip asks, "W-Where is John, our speech therapist friend and adviser?" Maura says, "The clinic here was reorganized and John left the university to work an hour away at a correctional institution. We miss seeing him and getting his clients as members." Phillip queries, "How about the guys from the military clinic? Are they still coming?" Ellen replies, "No. We do not see any guys from there anymore."

Lou stops at this point. Everyone is very appreciative of his summarizing the latest news. Everyone remarks that the national association seems to be very active with advocacy activities. Ellen comments that in the early 1970s they had educational activities to inform the public, professionals, and parents of children who stuttered but there were no assertive advocacy campaigns. "We-we have really dev-developed over the years, haven't haven't we," she said. Maura and Lou nodded their heads "yes"—"I'm really proud of how far we have come!" said Phillip.

Phillip wants to add some news from the West Coast. He says: "I w-went to the American Speech and Hearing Association [ASHA] meeting. The American Stuttering Program [ASP] had a booth jointly with your group. I sat in on the delib-deliberations with the officers of your group and ASP about wh-whether we should merge the two national organizations. Both sides were willing to compromise—you-you know ASP doesn't like us to be called stutterers and I guess your officers did not like the word 'program.' But they wondered how they would ever get together with the high airfares and all. They-they haven't decided anything yet."

"ASP membership, you know, is individuals, not groups," continues Phillip. Lou interjects that he is a member mostly because of the great newsletter—the editor's literary and history background really makes a difference. Phillip continues, "Groups are regarded as kind of secondary in ASP because they come and go so quickly, I guess. ASP now has a definite format for its groups—for a group to be affiliated, they have to agree to use it. Meet every two weeks, not monthly. And the first half of the meeting is sharing experiences among everyone. The second half is public speaking exercises copied after Toastmasters. Of course only positive criticism and encouragement is allowed. I was frightened to speak for three minutes without any preparation, but I'm getting over my fears gradually." Ellen asks Phillip, "Have you heard of the third national group for people who stutter that is here on the East Coast? It was started about six years ago; it's composed of groups, not individuals. The head of it and his wife attend our national conventions."

Maura announces in closing the meeting that they will continue their practice of having meetings once a month because attendance is down. Not enough people are willing to do the work to recruit new members—it seems as if the Caring Group is running out of energy.

"Is anyone interested in coffee after the meeting?" Phillip asks. Only Ellen wants to catch up with her old friend over coffee. At the coffee shop, Ellen confides that "our local group is falling apart. In fact, I think an ASP group is starting up in the suburbs but we sure aren't any competition. The old-timers mostly went on to accept new challenges in the regular world of fluent speakers. It's just Dick and me primarily who are still involved from those of the early 1970s. But Dick hardly ever comes to this meeting, preoccupied as he is with the national and even the international level—he's met people from groups in Scandinavia, England, Japan. We have no new blood. I'm getting tired of the same old topics, and being editor of the national newsletter is enough for me."

"But how did this happen?" Phillip asks. Ellen answers, "Did you hear about the group splitting off last year?" No, Phillip had not heard of it. Ellen continues, explaining that Carol and a group of people who had recently gone through Hollins College precision fluency shaping therapy had left to form a "maintenance therapy" group where they could practice the fluency they learned. "Isn't that the therapy that produces very slow monotone speech, with no emotion?" Phillip queries. "Yes," Ellen replies, "I personally couldn't stand it." Phillip and Ellen finish their coffee, asking the whereabouts of mutual friends. As they part, they agree to stay in touch regardless of the fate of the group for people who stutter.

Epilogue, 1998

Fifteen years later, the world of people who stutter has changed extensively. The National Caring Group for People Who Stutter dwindled away by the late 1980s; no groups are left. A single yearly conference, smaller and smaller, is their only activity. Now members of the ASP prop up the conference.

As the ASP's membership swelled, it faced organizational issues in the mid-1990s as its original leadership structure and procedures were inappropriate for the larger organization. Leadership changes were made. The ASP's focus on individuals as members rather than groups is fortuitous. If a national organization's members are groups, not individuals, then when a group folds, the national organization is likely to lose the individual members that were part of that group. If an individual discontinues membership, the loss is only one.

The Internet has significantly changed the world of contacts and information dissemination among professionals, groups for people who stutter, and individuals who stutter.

National and international contacts have led to the development of new networks, international conferences, and other forms of information exchange in an ever-widening spiral. An interesting story remains to be written about the changing terrain for people who stutter: from the "huddle together" group of the 1950s from which Joseph Sheehan distanced himself; through the 1970s and 1980s when the Caring Group evolved, transforming itself and assisting other self-help groups to form; to the 1980s and later when national-level self-help/mutual aid organizations have solidly established themselves. In the new millennium, global exchanges and networks are likely to be the next challenge.

| Chapter 6 | A Liberating Meaning Perspective |

THE STORY of the life cycle of the Caring Group on Stuttering over its seventeen years of existence was told in compressed form in the last chapter. Here, the story will be interpreted from an analytical framework in order to show how the group evolved a liberating meaning perspective. Simultaneously, the organizational structure evolved, and its relationship (or lack of relationship) to the meaning perspective will be charted.

The story of the Caring Group on Stuttering is special and distinctive. It was the first group of people who stutter to develop a liberating meaning perspective in the United States. Other groups may have been developing liberating meaning perspectives in the late 1960s and early 1970s in Sweden, Holland, New Zealand, Japan, and Finland, where we know strong and effective self-help groups existed (Borkman 1974), but we have no information about their meaning perspectives. By the 1970s other groups were formed in the United States, including the American Stuttering Program and Talk Comfortably.

Developing a Liberating Meaning Perspective

People with stigmatized conditions need a liberating meaning perspective that can free them of self-hate, a negative self-identity, and assumptions that they are inadequate. They need to redefine their humanity. Moreover, they need a constructive way of dealing with their problem.

A self-help/mutual aid commons exists in part to create a social space where people can freely define and evolve their own meanings and identity with regard to their shared problem, apart from the social groups or society that is devaluing them. From a societal standpoint, such commons can be incubators of social innovation and experimentation, although self-helpers probably begin not with the idea of innovating but with the goal of diminishing their pain and suffering.

The task of constructing a meaningful perspective that is practical and workable from the member's point of view is a social process occurring over a period of time. The literature on self-help groups rarely recognizes, much less studies, the stages of development groups undergo in evolving a meaning perspective, experiential authority, and an organizational structure. A three-stage process of the development of a group meaning perspective is presented for heuristic purposes. Empirical research may show that more or fewer stages need to be identified. I argue that the meaning perspective and experiential knowledge and authority develop in tandem, whereas the organizational structure may evolve independently. In discussing the three stages, the nature of the problem and its resolution, the social technology, and self-help identities will be detailed.

Consider a three-stage model of experiential development undergone by organizations: fledgling, developed, and mature (see table 6.1). The third-stage mature group can progress in one of two directions: open learning or closed and ossified.

The first stage is labeled "fledgling," a term that captures the uncertainty about the meaning and usefulness of their experiences that new groups face (G. Weber 1982). They may accept the authority of professional experts who are defining their problem and available solutions to a large extent. The group has no clear meaning perspective or frame of reference, and members are mired in their old negative identity. The members are likely to behave as victims. The structure of the group is likely to be informal and in the process of becoming organized.

Another type of fledgling group is the new group that has borrowed a meaning perspective from a nationally federated or affiliated group but has not undergone the learning process to apply the borrowed meaning perspective to itself and to make it its own. In chapter 5, the group for people who stutter was in the fledgling stage of development in 1966 during its first year. Members relied extensively on the authority of the professional speech therapist who sponsored the group and provided various resources to it. They shared experiences with one another and began to sift and sort out commonalities as part of the process of developing a workable definition of and resolution to their problem.

Table 6.1
Stages of Experiential Development of Groups

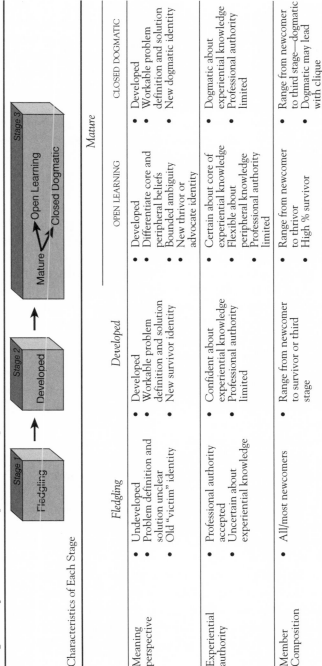

Characteristics of Each Stage

	Fledgling	Developed	Mature	
			OPEN LEARNING	CLOSED DOGMATIC
Meaning perspective	• Undeveloped • Problem definition and solution unclear • Old "victim" identity	• Developed • Workable problem definition and solution • New survivor identity	• Developed • Differentiate core and peripheral beliefs • Bounded ambiguity • New thrivor or advocate identity	• Developed • Workable problem definition and solution • New dogmatic identity
Experiential authority	• Professional authority accepted • Uncertain about experiential knowledge	• Confident about experiential knowledge • Professional authority limited	• Certain about core of experiential knowledge • Flexible about peripheral knowledge • Professional authority limited	• Dogmatic about experiential knowledge • Professional authority limited
Member Composition	• All/most newcomers	• Range from newcomer to survivor or third stage	• Range from newcomer to thrivor • High % survivor	• Range from newcomer to third stage—dogmatic • Dogmatic may lead with clique
Organizational issues	• Informal • Lack of norms/procedures • Leaders and positions unclear	• Organized • Structural form varies (12-step group, nonprofit bureaucracy)	• Bounded flexibility, stable • Structural form varies (12-step group, nonprofit bureaucracy)	• Rigidly stable • Structural form varies (12-step group, nonprofit bureaucracy)

The second stage is labeled "developed." At this stage a workable meaning perspective has been fashioned, which has given the group some confidence or experiential authority in the validity of its perspective. As members own their experiential wisdom, the authority they grant to professionals is lessened. A developed group is likely to have been in operation for some time. It has a number of old-timers or veterans who possess self-authority about its experiential knowledge. A developed commons is likely to have a range of members who vary in their extent of experiential understanding; importantly, the group has at least a strong minority of members who know and practice its framework in their daily lives. The longer-term and middle-term members maintain the group's culture, pass on the knowledge to newcomers through their sharing, and manifest their knowledge in the way they live their lives.

The group is likely to be organized, but the structure can take one of several forms: 12-step group, nonprofit collectivist organization, or nonprofit bureaucratic organization. The group for people who stutter was a developed group by 1971. The open-minded speech therapist adviser still provided some resources, but the group was governing its own affairs and making its own operating rules. It had a workable liberating meaning perspective. It was well organized with a basic hierarchical nonprofit structure.

The third stage is labeled "mature" and can take at least two forms: an open learning group or a closed dogmatic group. The open learning group has evolved beyond confidence into certainty about the central core of its beliefs that need to be maintained; peripheral beliefs can be changed to adapt to the environment. Members include some thrivors or advocates (the third stage for individuals) who lead the group. The Caring Group was in the third stage by 1976. The closed dogmatic group has an alternative position of certainty, having evolved beyond confidence. However, the dogmatic group displays experiential authority about its entire perspective, rather than differentiating between core and peripheral beliefs as does the open learning group. For the dogmatic group, the meaning perspective is largely fixed, and the group believes that it has the "truth" about solving its problem. The leaders are likely to be the orthodox, sometimes a clique of the orthodox and their followers. The structure can vary from an "ossified" 12-step group to a nonprofit bureaucracy.

Empirical research may show a different number of stages than the three suggested here or different characteristics for a stage.[1] Groups, like individuals, do not necessarily or inevitably go through all these stages. Some can remain in the first or second stage indefinitely or disband after the first or second stage. Some can jump from the fledgling stage to the third stage, especially the closed dogmatic version.

FLEDGLING: CARING GROUP ON STUTTERING

The original attendees to the group were primarily stuttering clients of the speech therapist John, who helped cofound the group and became its adviser. His participation was critical in the beginning to provide

1. the beginnings of a meaning perspective: the nonavoidance philosophy,
2. his professional authority about the appropriateness and workability of the meaning perspective and the organizational approach,
3. organizational skill in how to operate a group and to teach others how to operate such a group, and
4. resources, including a meeting place, a mailing address, and a source of potential members whom he referred from his clients.

The societal context in which a self-help group evolves significantly affects the perspectives and knowledge available about the problem of interest, as well as the institutions, professions, and organizations that have staked a claim on defining and treating/intervening in resolving the problem. Self-helpers are aware of the ways their problem is viewed by various audiences in society.

Stuttering is stigmatized or subjected to penalizing social reactions to varying degrees depending upon the social context, culture, status, and listener. Most adults who stutter are part-time normal speakers, which tempts them to project a social identity as a fluent speaker and makes it even more difficult to accept the nonavoidance approach of deliberately and openly stuttering in social interaction. But, paradoxically, in avoiding stuttering, the person develops facial and bodily movements associated with trying to speak that makes her speaking behavior more observable to the listener (Petrunik 1974, 202).

Many adults who stutter feel inadequate as human beings partly because of their social identity as a person who stutters and their personal experiences of having been rejected and ridiculed, and having so often elicited negative reactions from listeners. Many attendees at the Caring Group were seeing and hearing other people who stuttered for the first time. The attendees were primarily working and middle class, many young college students or professionals with solid work histories.

In the 1960s and 1970s (and up to the present), as noted in chapter 5, a multitude of theories existed about the causes and treatment of stuttering. Was the problem slow disfluent speech and the mechanisms of talking? Or was it a broader communication problem that included far more than the mechanics of speaking, such as one's interaction with listeners, nonverbal communication, and one's self-concept? Was stuttering caused by defective physiological mechanisms of speech, inadequacy of personality, or something else?

Many stuttering therapies were available, although the field of speech pathology as a whole may have been largely indifferent to the problem of stuttering, and no institutionalized professional treatment was sanctioned. Folk notions about curing stuttering abounded, as did commercial remedies that promised relief but were largely expensive and useless. The nonavoidance approach to stuttering was taught by John to the group as the best available way of defining and resolving stuttering. The manner in which a group frames the definition of the problem affects the possible solutions. Stuttering was defined as a chronic, that is life-long, intermittent, and presently incurable condition. Interestingly, a few dual-status professionals (speech therapists or psychologists who were recovered stutterers), such as Dr. Joseph Sheehan and Dr. Charles Van Riper, had developed this abstract, complex, but liberating approach. The fact that the developers of the nonavoidance approach were recovered stutterers probably increased its credibility to members of the Caring Group.[2]

The attendees of the group accepted John's professional authority that validated the nonavoidance approach. However, they had to experience it for themselves and work with it until they could own it. There were major problems with the nonavoidance approach. It was extemely abstract, paradoxical, and demanding. It appeared to create new problems as it allegedly solved others. Its abstract nature was a serious impediment, for how did one translate it into daily activities that one could practice to learn to behave differently? Its thesis was counterintuitive and went against common sense: admit you stutter, and the more open you are about being a person who stutters, the less disfluent you will be. Paradoxically, you more visibly reveal the broken speech that is stigmatized and elicits negative reactions from some listeners. Moreover, the approach's premise that stuttering is presently incurable was unacceptable to many people. The complexity of the stuttering problem and the bewildering array of theories and therapies made the development of a workable meaning perspective more difficult than for some problems.

Analogous conditions today to stuttering in the 1960s are eating disorders. Science is reporting breakthroughs in the genetics and physiological mechanisms of eating disorders. Overweight people can choose among many folk ideas regarding the solution to overeating as well as those found in popular magazines. They may also choose among medical practitioners who specialize in eating disorders, self-help groups (for example, Overeaters Anonymous or TOPS–Take Off Pounds Sensibly), or corporate support groups (such as Weight Watchers) or other for-profit plans to lose weight (such as Jenny Craig). Or they can reject societal norms of slimness and join an advocacy group such as Fat Is Beautiful.

In contrast to stuttering in the 1960s and overeating today, when Alcoholics Anonymous was founded in 1935, health professionals were uninterested in alcohol problems, and they were defined more as a moral defect than an illness. Alcoholics were usually found in jails or mental hospitals or in the gutter. No professionalized alcohol treatment industry existed that either needed to maintain its turf or was promoting its own view of alcoholism. The alcoholic thus had few avenues to try. Furthermore, a relatively simple solution was found to work: abstinence from alcohol (although maintaining abstinence became the long-term challenge). The alcoholics in early AA groups had few competing ideas about alcoholism or its treatment to test like the people who stutter did.

When it began in 1966, the Caring Group on Stuttering had many avenues to explore, test, and eliminate in order to find a satisfactory solution to its members' stuttering problem. During the fledgling stage between 1966 and 1969, the group held discussions—the circle of sharing—to identify which aspects of stuttering members had in common, which issues associated with stuttering were problematic such as talking on the telephone, and which techniques they used to cope with these difficulties. This early phase of identifying grievances and problems has been called the "Speak Bitterness" phase of consciousness raising; the Speak Bitterness phase is disproportionately composed of the whining that some critics mistake as the whole (Borkman 1975a). In part members were identifying both their strategies to avoid stuttering and their experiences with various forms of treatment and its outcomes.

Newcomers wanted, wished for, and expected to find a cure for their stuttering, something that would give them fluency. The idea that a "cure" is attainable if one looks hard enough or wants one badly enough is alive and well in modern culture; some attendees who came a few times and did not return were disappointed to learn the group did not expect to find a cure to their stuttering (Borkman 1976).

In the early years, the leaders and seasoned members seemed to define the nature of their problem fairly narrowly as a speech disorder rather than more broadly as a communication disorder involving self-concept, relationship to listener, and so forth. They focused on stuttering therapies that emphasized the mechanics of speech, even though the nonavoidance philosophy implied that it was a broader communication disorder.

The discovery learning process proceeds somewhat as follows: if you think you are the only one who has had stuttering therapy (or worse yet, several therapies) but it stopped working, you are likely to blame yourself for resuming stuttering. However, when you discuss the issue with peers who stutter, and you hear of case after case of similar situations with the same consequences (that is, stuttering therapy eliminates stuttering for a while, then the person resumes stuttering), then you question your earlier conclusion, namely, that it is your fault the therapy stopped working. When you view your peers as reasonable people—intelligent, educated, competent, motivated, and problem solving—and they have experiences similar to yours, then you are likely to question your premises and assumptions.

SOCIAL TECHNOLOGY. "Technology" refers to that part of the meaning perspective in which the group process—the relationships among participants or tasks—is used as and regarded as part of the intervention to resolve the problem. To what extent are the relationships among participants designed or thought about as part of the "recovery process" for individuals or as facilitating goal achievement? In 12-step groups, the 12 steps, which are guidelines for individual recovery, are part of the technology as well as the 12 traditions, which are guidelines for maintenance of the group. Irving Gellman (1964), who made an early organizational analysis of AA, talked about the dynamics of local AA groups as constituting "organizational therapy." The social technology could include aspects of the group process (for example, the circle of sharing, or additional goals beyond helping members, or friendship/community building) that are designed to facilitate members' learning, healing, and recovery.

The safe sharing circle is a major social technology of the Caring Group. The activity of everyone saying his or her name out loud at the end of the meeting has been routinized as part of the technology. Probably the most difficult speaking task for most adults who stutter is saying their name out loud. The custom was instituted because it is so difficult and because it would therefore be "therapeutic" to diminish the fear of saying one's name.

Another part of its initial social technology was the idea that friendships and social events outside the meetings could cause it to deteriorate into a whining "huddle-together" group and were therefore dangerous. This unfortunate idea deterred the group from having social events and from striking up friendships to some extent, but over time some became friends in and around group activities with seemingly no ill effects, and the validity of the idea began to be questioned.

IDENTITY. The issue of how one's identity was tied to stuttering emerged as important in the early years of the group. Members grew to realize that they had negative personal identities as a result of their stuttering and that their stuttering identity had become a "master status" that engulfed their identities; that is, they defined themselves as if stuttering was the primary characteristic that affected everything else about them (Becker 1963). They also began to see that a positive self-identity was possible as they admired one another as "normal competent adults" and found that many members were creative and possessed many skills, including being able to keep their organization operating. Sally expressed relief in the early 1966 meeting at seeing attendees who were "normal looking and accomplished people."

Karen Yoshida (1998) has formulated ideas about the reshaping of selves that adults with traumatic spinal cord injury undergo that also apply to many other conditions for which self-help groups are formed. She views the process of recovery as a pendulum that swings back and forth, in which an individual vacillates with respect to which view of his self predominates, even on a daily basis. Five selves are pertinent:

1. The former self, or the normal person before the trauma (which does not apply to adults who stutter, as most of them began stuttering in early childhood, but it does apply to other self-helpers),
2. The "disabled identity as the total self," a negative identity,
3. The "disabled identity as part of the total self" (with realistic recognition of limitations imposed by the disability),
4. The "supernormal identity," where the person engages in activities of an extraordinary nature and will not ask for assistance, and
5. The "middle self," who is realistic about limitations but sees herself as more than the disability and has developed a "collective disabled consciousness" in which there is wider social concern for other persons with the disability. The middle self is the point in the pendulum between the extreme supernormal identity on the one hand and the "disabled identity as the total self" at the other extreme.

Many attendees generalized from a negative social identity to a negative personal identity. For example, Sally expressed a negative identity in being relieved to see that people who stutter were not black sheep or oddballs in the 1966 meeting. Many newcomers to the group attribute all their problems to the fact that they stutter. Attributing all their problems to stuttering is an illustration of Yoshida's "disabled as total identity." Or they infer causality incorrectly; in the 1967 meeting that dealt with the outcomes of their previous attempts at speech therapy, some inferred that something was wrong with them because they could not carry over fluency from the therapist's office to their daily life. During the sharing circle process, in which a number of people are found to have had similar negative experiences, these incorrect inferences can be identified and changed.

An interesting case is Tom, the fluent person with a self-identity as stutterer, in the 1969 meeting. He does not have any speaking issues, but he has the self-concept of a stutterer that is his total identity. This identity keeps him from risking new activities of living.[3]

NATURE OF THE PROBLEM AND ITS RESOLUTION. By 1971, five years after initiation, a liberating meaning perspective had been constructed by the seasoned members and old-timers of the Caring Group. Newcomers who came in wanting to find a cure had to go through the process of coming to accept the nonavoidance approach for themselves, or they did not return. Some seasoned members left the group in keeping with the norm that the expected duration of membership was several years: once members were comfortable with their stuttering, some would join the fluent world.

Some original members, especially those who became officers and assumed other leadership positions in the Caring Group, tested the nonavoidance approach in their lives. From John's speech therapy they got help with the mechanics of stuttering to stutter more comfortably. As they took advantage of the speaking opportunities involved in the external goals of educating parents about their children's stuttering or informing speech therapists about their Caring Group, they talked more and learned to stop avoiding stuttering. They found that the paradoxes were true: the more they were open about stuttering, the less severe were their blocks. In the process of taking speaking risks and learning to stutter more comfortably, they gained experiential authority about what they were doing. For example, in the 1971 meeting Ralph and Joe review another form of speech therapy and critique it; they know they are knowledgeable enough from their own and other members' experiences to evaluate the likely result of the proposed speech therapy. A commercial gimmick, the Edinburgh Masker, is also described in a meeting, and Phyllis explains that, yes, it works, but with speech at an unnatural cadence. The group is distinguishing among different types of fluency and developing values about what kind of speech they want. John, their adviser, still maintains his authority in their eyes because of his broad knowledge of speech pathology and therapies, but they had developed their own self-authority as a result of resolving their stuttering problems.

The respect for the attendee's preferences for type of speaking (fluency with cadence or monotone versus spontaneity and expressiveness with stuttering), type of speech therapy, or other forms of therapy is a value that has developed in the organization.

SOCIAL TECHNOLOGY. At the second stage the safe sharing circle is still the major social technology of the Caring Group. Assuming organizational responsibilities is also recognized to be important to recovery. In a leadership role a person has opportunities to speak and takes responsiblity for planning, organizing, and implementing events of the group.

IDENTITY. By this time a positive identity has been constructed, namely, that stuttering is but one of their characteristics and does not define them; furthermore, stuttering is not as negatively perceived as it was in 1966. Stuttering is seen as a mild disability that need not restrict their life chances or opportunities, unless they let it.

Testing the nonavoidance approach in their own lives and finding that the paradoxes were true, that when they were open, they stuttered less severely, has bolstered members' self-confidence and contributed to their positive identity. As they experiment with other activities in their lives and find other talents they possess, their identity swings to Yoshida's third self ("the disabled identity as part of the total self") or even to the desirable "middle self," in which the person acknowledges his or her stuttering as a minor limitation and has developed a "collective stuttering consciousness," as well as a concern about people who stutter. Officers and other leaders of the Caring Group who engage in external education and advocacy activities or organizational maintenance are especially likely to swing to the middle self.

THIRD STAGE: MATURE

NATURE OF PROBLEM AND ITS RESOLUTION. By 1976, ten years after founding, the Caring Group is in the third stage of development, a mature open learning group. New kinds of therapy are still considered by the group and evaluated on the basis of their collective experience. They are much more discerning about what is potentially useful and what is a gimmick.

The group has broadened its perspective and views stuttering as a total communication disorder involving the mechanisms of speech, contact with the listener, the listener's reaction, and self-concept. In resolving one's stuttering problem, changing one's perspective about the significance of the problem in one's life is key. With stuttering, the process involves diminishing the impact of that piece of identity on the whole. But the group has had to learn it together over a long period of time in order to pass it on to its members. In AA and with other addictions, in contrast, denial or the inability to recognize the problem and its impact on one's life means that self-helpers have to change their perspective to an understanding that their addiction is a major issue affecting all aspects of their life.

SOCIAL TECHNOLOGY. In the third stage the sharing circle is still a mainstay of the group's technology but it has limited appeal for seasoned members because topics are often repeated over a several-year period. The sharing circle is especially useful for newcomers, but some more advanced form of "talking activity" is needed for the seasoned members. No other stimulating or more advanced talking activities have been introduced; Toastmasters was considered and rejected.

The openness of the Caring Group to new therapies is exhibited in the discussion of the precision shaping fluency program at Hollins College in the 1976 meeting. This therapy produces fluency with monotone speech, and again, different values about speaking are found among the attendees; diversity of opinion is respected.

The idea of Dr. Sheehan's that friendships and social events are problematic has dissipated through their experience of being friends with one another with no negative results. Members meet for coffee after meetings and have social events several times a year.

IDENTITY. An even more positive social identity has been fashioned than was found earlier; a person who stutters is a normal person with a slight defect. Furthermore, the idea has developed that a person who stutters has rights in public—such as the right to take the time needed to express what one wants in a retail situation. Ellen, for example, expressed self-advocacy, or standing up for her rights. Members who lead the group or help develop the national group exhibit a "middle self" in Yoshida's terms, in that they have a "collective conscience" concerning people who stutter and do advocacy work to help them.

Joe, a long-term member and several-time officer, has gone a step further in being open about his stuttering. At appropriate times in a new relationship he speaks directly with the other person about the fact that he does stutter. He and others have discovered that when they are not embarrassed or upset about disfluencies, the listener is unlikely to be discomforted either.

Organizational Issues

Voluntary organizations in the nonprofit and voluntary third sector operate in special ways owing to their distinctive natures. All purposively planned social collectivities have a number of problems to solve in order to maintain themselves. They need an adequate number of members, resources, goals or vision, leadership, and a program or means of working toward their vision. Wuthnow (1994) found that members of small groups (which included Bible study and Sunday school groups, self-help groups, and special interest groups) reported having a leader, purpose, agenda or schedule (regular time to meet), name, and elected officers as important minimal structures to group function-ing. All organizations need to find workable ways of motivating their mem-bers to follow the program and work toward achieving their vision or goals. Membership organizations such as self-help groups need to satisfy their mem-bers in order to maintain their participation and contribution to organizational maintenance.

MEMBERS

Charles Perrow (1970) has dissected the ways in which "members" can be re-garded as resources of voluntary associations. The member's name, money, personpower, or self (personality) may be valued as a major resource. For ex-ample, the American Association of Retired Persons (AARP) relies on its members' *names* and *money* in order to do its work; in lobbying Congress the organization adds up the number of names on its rolls to show its strength. Dues from millions of members finance many educational campaigns to Con-gress. AARP is run by professionals who make and implement the policy, of-ten with little concern about the members' personpower or self.

In contrast, true self-help groups rely primarily on their members' selves (personality) and secondarily their personpower; people's actual attendance, listening to and telling stories at meetings, is important for the group's func-tioning, as was described in the sharing circle in chapter 1. In addition, mem-bers' contributions of time and energy (personpower) to group projects as well as organizational maintenance activities are important to goal achievement and survival.

Some self-help networks rely on members as resources in terms of names and money instead of personpower and selves. Lone individuals pay dues to a national organization; the organization primarily operates in terms of a news-letter or other impersonal communication among members who may be wide-spread geographically. Members do not work on projects together other than letter-writing campaigns or the equivalent. Individuals relate to the central node of the network where the newsletter is produced; "Resources for People with Facial Difference," a newsletter published by Let's Face It, a group for people with "facial differences," is an example (Let's Face It 1997).

Resources of names or money are storable and transferable. Money can be used to buy other goods or services; names can be used as evidence of the quantity or quality of your membership. If one's resources are members as personpower or personalities, however, these are not storable or transferable. A person attends a meeting to help herself or to be an involved participant today. Tomorrow may be another matter. The self-help group that relies on members' personpower and personality has to continually be attractive to its potential membership in the here and now in order to elicit their voluntary participation. In that sense, self-help groups are "living organizations" in that they have perishable memberships that are here today but not necessarily tomorrow. Furthermore, they are "living organizations" in that the character of the group is greatly affected by the current composition of members, since they bring themselves (as their personality) and their personpower as the major resource to the organization. Therefore, even small changes in membership can affect the character and functioning of the group.

Organizations evolve expectations about how long members should continue participating, and what, if any, are members' obligations to contribute to organizational maintenance. Organizational maintenance involves a wide variety of tasks such as setting up meeting rooms, planning programs, chairing meetings, recruiting new members, making coffee or bringing refreshments, and maintaining members' interest.

The Caring Group on Stuttering developed the expectation that successful members would leave the group after several years in order to participate as "normal persons" in the wider fluent world. No clear-cut or consistent expectations evolved that members were obligated to help maintain the organization, although at points this message was conveyed by the officers. In fact, conflict sometimes surfaced over the issue of organizational maintenance. Maintainers, such as Ralph the attorney, helped the group become a legally incorporated nonprofit organization its first year. Other members, such as Ellen or Maria, did not regard time spent on organizational maintenance as important. Ironically, Ralph stayed in the group for about five years and then left entirely, whereas Ellen continued her contributions through the last fourteen years or so of the group's existence.

The Caring Group was a very open group, although there were restrictions on who could be an officer. Participants varied widely in how frequently they attended, the length of time they attended, and their degree of participation in the leadership or organizational maintenance of the commons. Long-term members were more likely to be officers, but occasionally a newcomer accepted a leadership role.

GOVERNANCE

Many adults who stutter avoid participation in voluntary associations because of their fear of talking, and thus they have had little or no experience in leading or maintaining organizations. The early leaders of the Caring Group thought that the conventional nonprofit organizational format with a hierarchy of a board, officers, and members would provide clear positions or opportunities for members to develop leadership skills. They recognized the importance of providing situations for members to develop organizational expertise.

Later, in the 1980s, when two national organizations for people who stutter, the American Stuttering Program and the National Caring Group, were considering merging into one national organization, they decided against the merger. One reason given was the issue of leadership opportunities: one national organization would provide fewer leadership positions for people who stutter to gain skills.

The Caring Group developed its organizational structure and process during its first year. By the 1967 meeting described in chapter 5 it had a constitution and bylaws and was legally incorporated as a nonprofit organization. John, the fluent therapist, was allowed to be an officer during the first years, but the bylaws were changed in 1971 and allowed only people who stutter to be officers. The charter specified an advisory board composed of professionals that could recommend actions for the board but could not make decisions. This formalized organizational format developed so quickly largely because the leader Ralph was a lawyer who was interested in applying his knowledge and legal expertise to help the group without charge.

Some other important aspects of the organizational structure are questions of the openness of the membership of the group—does it include family members of those with the problem, professionals specializing in this problem, and other interested persons? The Caring Group was open to family members and professional speech therapists whether they stuttered or not. For example, Ned, the father of a young person who stuttered, visited the 1966 meeting, and speech therapists visited in 1967.

ROLE OF PROFESSIONALS AND AGENCIES

John, who sponsored the group, provided extensive guidance and leadership during the first years until the cofounders and other officers had developed more leadership skills and experience. John can be characterized as a "normal-smith." An extremely open, self-help-friendly professional, he from the beginning did not want the group to be dependent upon him but appropriately coached the officers to develop necessary organizational skills. John's role as normal-smith, imputing normality to people who stuttered and regarding them with respect and admiration, was important. Lofland (1969) maintains that normal-smiths are critical to people who have been labeled undesirably different (or as social deviants), because the tendency in society is to assume that people cannot change: once a stutterer, always a stutterer.

The role of the professional speech therapist in the group changed over time. In 1966, when the group was founded, the therapist cofounded and then sponsored the group. He obtained resources from his university clinic such as a meeting room and mailing address, provided direction on organizational issues, and articulated a meaning perspective from his professional colleagues that was the basis of the liberating one the group developed. His clients in stuttering therapy provided a source of members. He developed and led projects with the group such as the writing and taping of a television script. By the mid-1970s, John attended meetings infrequently, becoming more of a sympathizer. He was available behind the scenes for advice or help on special organizational problems. As the Caring Group became more autonomous, John focused his efforts on helping other self-help groups for adults who stutter to organize following the format of the Caring Group. By the early 1980s John took another job with a long commute outside the city and was no longer at the clinic where the group's meetings were held. He became in effect a "friend of the group" at that point. At the same time the university closed the speech and hearing clinic. The Caring Group then had to negotiate meeting space with the new center, since it had no personal relationships with any center staff that would ease the negotiation process.

RESOURCE DEPENDENCE

The Caring Group was moderately dependent on resources. Recuiting members' personpower and personalities, material aid (meeting room and mailing address), professional ideas and interventions (such as the nonavoidance approach to stuttering, stuttering speech therapy), and organizational development skills were needed. Over time sufficient Caring Group members developed organizational skills to maintain the organization, though not without fits and starts (in 1967, for example, all the officers were asked to resign as they had been inactive). By or before 1976, members were running the organization essentially by themselves.

The Caring Group retained its dependence on external sources for recruiting members. In the 1960s, adults who stuttered were scattered throughout the population and did not know or interact with one another; potential members were located through speech therapists who specialized in treating stuttering. For a number of years the Caring Group had a ready supply of potential members from John and then from a nearby military speech clinic, which referred potential members between the late 1960s and mid-1970s.

By 1980 neither the military clinic nor John was sending potential members to the Caring Group. By its demise in 1983, the organizationally strong leaders had left the Caring Group because of their success in living in the fluent world (such as Joe, Ralph, and Stan) or they turned their attention to broader arenas of national and international self-help (such as Dick and Ellen).

The isolation of people who stutter has changed somewhat in the 1990s. The activities of three national organizations since the 1970s, yearly conventions that draw members from all three organizations, and the Internet have created a loose national network. The Internet is allowing an international network of people who stutter to evolve.

GOALS AND VALUES

The major goals and values subscribed to by members are an important part of a commons, since they are often founded in order to express and realize certain values.[4] In legally incorporated nonprofit organizations, the goals are explicitly written but general in form; in more informal groups they may be unwritten. Both the internal goals, benefiting members of the group, and the external goals are important. External goals in this story might include: (1) helping others who stutter, (2) educating the public or professionals, or (3) advocacy to reduce discrimination against people who stutter.

The major activities and focus of the Caring Group were internally oriented to its members; this internal orientation was reflected in the basic meeting format, the sharing circle. However, the group also had important secondary external goals of educating the families of those who stutter, especially children who stutter, and the public about the disorder. In addition, the group added advocacy goals in the mid-1970s.

The group usually had some activity oriented toward achieving its external goals of education, as is seen in the announcements at the beginning of meetings in 1967, 1969, 1971, and 1976. The external activities also benefited members, since they involved speaking opportunities (and were part of their methodology of problem resolution) such as public workshops, television shows about stuttering, or sponsoring a booth about their group at the American Speech and Hearing Association convention.

As the Caring Group evolved its liberating perspective, values about options for kind of fluency or approach to stuttering were identified and clarified. For example, the Edinburgh Masker was a gimmick that produced fluency but with a cadence, as described in the 1971 meeting; similarly precision fluency shaping was a form of speech therapy described in the 1976 meeting that produced fluency with a monotone. Members had different opinions about the importance of fluency relative to spontaneous emotionally expressive speech.

INFORMAL ORGANIZATION AND COMMUNITY

Informal organization, that is, a network of personal and social relationships among members, is a ubiquitous part of viable organizations.[5] The informal organization is the connective tissue that allows the formal organization to work; co-workers go to lunch, celebrate special occasions, become friends or lovers, exchange gifts, and the like. These relationships establish trust, familiarity, and common understandings that facilitate the completion of formal or planned activities. In a voluntary association, the member's motivation to attend and contribute to organizational maintenance depends importantly on the network of personal and social relationships he or she develops with other participants. Work organizations use incentives such as salaries, fringe benefits, or prestige, but these utilitarian rewards are minimal in the commons.

In the Caring Group on Stuttering, the therapist sponsor warned members in 1966 against holding social events or developing friendships outside of meetings, and the group initially followed that advice. Over time, as members became friends, they saw that the more involved they were with one another inside and outside meetings, the more personal progress they made. They tested the idea experientially that fraternizing was harmful and rejected it as untrue. They began having parties and forming friendships before 1971. By 1976 they met regularly after the meetings for coffee or beer. The social events, which often included their families, continued over the lifespan of the group.

Why was Joseph Sheehan incorrect in his presumption that friendships and social events were producing the inward-looking "huddle-together" group? Other reasons may explain why his group developed as it did. His group apparently had no external goals or activities that would have broadened members' focus beyond themselves. Although Sheehan presumably helped teach group participants the nonavoidance approach because they had been his clients in stuttering therapy, they were unable to create a liberating perspective. Furthermore, it appears that they received little help in developing organizational skills. The net result of no external goals or activities, no liberating standpoint, and weak organizational skills was that their friendships reinforced their avoidance of stuttering and of the fluent world. Just the reverse was true of the Caring Group, whose friendships reinforced its members' external orientation, facilitated the evolution of the liberating meaning perspective, and fostered the development of organizational skills.

THE CARING GROUP'S ENDING: FAILURE OR COMMUNITY RESOURCE?
The timing of the demise of the Caring Group as a separate organization may be unknowable. After it split in two in the 1980s owing to the different values of the proponents of the precision fluency shaping program and the regular members, it withered away over a period of time. At the 1983 meeting described in chapter 5 there were only three local attendees and one out-of-town visitor. Although the group still had scheduled meetings, sometimes only

one or two people showed up, as Ellen confided to the visitor Phillip over coffee. The loss of membership when the Hollins College therapy proponents left the group, combined with the lack of leadership and the lack of recruitment to find more members, left the Caring Group with reduced viability. When the group actually disbanded is unclear.

How do we interpret the ending of the Caring Group on Stuttering? Conventional organizational theory, especially the population ecology version that considers the rise and fall of classes of organizations in relation to the needs of a sector, would classify it as a failure. Recently, the issue of viewing the disbanding of voluntary organizations as failure has been questioned. In the early 1970s, for example, members of a New Zealand group for people who stutter decided to discontinue their self-help group because it had satisfied their needs. Especially for membership organizations that are constructed specifically for the good of their members, the idea that they can decide to dissolve the organization makes sense. Disbanding may connote success, not failure.[6]

An alternative perspective from a broader societal viewpoint is that although the organization per se has dissolved, the community is left enriched because the members have gained organizational skills, knowledge, self-confidence, and so forth. Carl Milofsky (1987, 1988) takes a broad community perspective of voluntary groups; he suggests that although a specific group disbanded, the community maintains the experience, skills, and knowledge gained from the group since its members continue to reside in the community. These resources are then available and are likely to be used for some future voluntary enterprise. New voluntary organizations will arise that are more suited for the needs of the community at that time, and the previous members can contribute to the new venture. Thus, from a community viewpoint, the pool of talent and human resources has increased even though one less organization exists.

When one takes a long-term perspective of half a century, one sees major increases in human resources for helping adults who stutter in the United States. A few attempts at starting a self-help group in the 1950s were failures. My study of self-help groups in the early 1970s found a somewhat more encouraging picture. A number of groups existed that were helping their members, according to their self-reports, although at that time groups without speech therapists or professional involvement did not survive. Normal-smiths, especially John from the Caring Group, directly helped five groups and indirectly helped three groups to organize between 1966 and 1971. The pool of stuttering adults who gained confidence in public speaking and developed other organizational skills increased. By the late 1970s three national self-help/ mutual aid organizations for people who stutter had developed; yearly conferences were held by the three organizations and a network was developing. By

the early 1980s, in a study of thirty-seven self-help organizations for people
who stutter, groups with a speech therapist were less likely to survive than in
1973; enough adults who stuttered had organizational skills or the confidence
that they could develop them (Borkman, Shaw, Shaw, and Hickey 1984).

Implications for Self-Help/Mutual Aid Commons

The story of the Caring Group raises general organizational issues about the
development of meaning perspectives, experiential authority, and organizational structures.

The diversity of meaning perspectives among self-help groups is extensive, as indicated by the typology described in chapter 1. Among other things,
groups vary in:

1. the domains (areas of the problem and its resolution) explicitly included
   as part of experiential knowledge or as requiring technical professional
   knowledge and outside the purview of experiential knowledge, and
2. the openness of the group to participants with different worldviews and
   different demographic and other characteristics.

A facet of the framework concerning the nature of stuttering is the beliefs about what are the life domains and situations the stuttering problem affects. From the beginning of the Caring Group in 1966, the idea that their
stuttering affected them physically, mentally, emotionally, and socially was
present. The spiritual domain was never explicitly included in the group's
framework, although individuals such as Ellen did in private; she confides at
the coffee shop after the 1976 meeting that she feels she has received a spiritual gift of grace from the love and understanding she receives in the Caring
Group.

The domains—or areas of the problem definition and resolution—regarded as accessible to experiential knowledge as well as those aspects regarded
as technical and so requiring professional knowledge vary from group to group.
In my study of three self-help groups—AA, the group for people who stutter,
and an ostomy association—the most obvious difference in domains was the
12-step AA group's inclusion of the spiritual as an integral part of the problem and resolution (Borkman 1979). The other two groups, which were organized as nonprofit hierarchies, excluded the spiritual from their framework.
The three groups also varied in terms of which aspects of their problem were
regarded as requiring professional knowledge. The ostomy association depended
so heavily on physicians and nurses to resolve its members' problem that professional knowledge was part of the accepted authority in the group. The group

for people who stutter varied over time in how reliant it was on the professional authority of the speech therapist to define the problem of stuttering and its resolution as described earlier in this chapter. Members began with no experiential knowledge of their own, but within five years they had grown largely independent of the speech therapist's authority. The AA group was the most developed of the three groups in relying on the experiential knowledge of its recovering members, although it recognized that the medical complications of alcoholism should be treated by a physician and that many members require outside counseling or therapy.

The openness of the group to minority ethnic and racial members, working- or lower-class members, the disabled, or those of differing lifestyles is frequently raised (T. Powell 1994). Although observers claim that some groups are hospitable only to a narrow range of demographic profiles, in fact there are only limited empirical data on which to base conclusions. Observations may be biased by the demographics of the observer who attends only certain kinds of groups in certain locations and inappropriately generalizes (Humphreys and Woods 1994). International studies of AA show that there is extensive demographic and worldview variation within a nation like the United States as well as cross-culturally (Caetano 1993; Makela 1993).

The fit between the group and participants with varying worldviews, demographic characteristics, and so on—in K. I. Maton's ecological framework (1993), the person-group fit—needs further research. A few studies touch upon this issue (Antze 1976; Medvene et al. 1994). For example, Louis Medvene and associates (1994) found that Mexican-American parents with a newly diagnosed mentally ill child were less likely to attend NAMI (National Alliance for the Mentally Ill) meetings if they thought their child's behavior was a moral defect, not an illness. How close a match between the elements of a framework and the participant's worldview is needed for attendance at a group over time? What kinds of incompatibilities result in participants' leaving the group? Are there differences among participants' capacity to "take what they want" of the group's framework "and leave the rest"? These and other questions need to be researched in a variety of groups.[7]

The "teachings of a group are its essence," says Paul Antze (1976, 324). In contrast with groups that are evolving a meaning perspective like the Caring Group, established groups such as Alcoholics Anonymous have codified their perspective into a general template or guide for others to follow. A template, a pattern or gauge used as a guide to the form of a work, has the same four components as a meaning perspective, but it is codified and relatively easily transferred to and adapted by other groups. The template of Alcoholics

Anonymous is the 12-steps, 12 traditions, and the ideas in the first 164 pages of the book *Alcoholics Anonymous*, also referred to as the "Big Book" ([1939] 1976), and the book known as the "12 and 12," or *Twelve Steps and Twelve Traditions* (Alcoholics Anonymous [1952] 1974).

The history of how the template developed in AA is well documented in Ernest Kurtz's *Not God* (1979). An indicator of the workability of AA's template is the fact that it has been borrowed by one hundred or more 12-step anonymous groups, with the permission of AA. Such groups as Debtors Anonymous, Gamblers Anonymous, Al-Anon, and Overeaters Anonymous borrow the AA template, adapting it for their own issue. Typically a new 12-step group will slightly rewrite the 12 steps and 12 traditions, substituting its issue for "alcohol" or "alcoholism." New groups often use the AA "Big Book" as part of their official literature. The 12 steps of AA are widely recognized to be important parts of its teachings or meaning perspective, but the 12 traditions, the principles guiding the group, are no less important. The significance of the 12 traditions will be shown in chapter 8, which analyzes AA as a self-organizing learning organization; organizational learning theory explores how some organizations successfully "learn," or change and adapt, while others do not.

The Caring Group on Stuttering took about ten years to develop its liberating perspective in its complete form; it developed its group process within a year or two, but the other elements took longer. In contrast, Alcoholics Anonymous had developed its frame for the definition of the problem, its resolution, and its identity within four years of its founding in 1935, with the publication of *Alcoholics Anonymous* in 1939. AA's meaning perspective for organizational processes, the 12 traditions, took much longer; they first appeared in the AA magazine *The Grapevine* in April 1946. Both AA and the Caring Group borrowed ideas from others in developing their meaning perspective (see Kurtz 1979 for the history of AA). Among other ideas, AA adapted ideas from the Oxford Group as part of its 12 steps; the Caring Group borrowed the nonavoidance approach from professional speech therapists. In these and other cases, the ideas borrowed from others are adapted, tested for workability, and refined to fit the circumstances of the group.

The differing experiences of the Caring Group and AA indicate that the organizational issues may be decided on a different time schedule than the other components of the framework. The histories of AA and the Caring Group on Stuttering also indicate that there is no set time order in which the components evolve.

Factors that are likely to affect the process or length of time of evolution of a meaning perspective include: the nature and characteristics of the problem, the social, cultural, and institutional context, the number and composition of members who test the frame, the degree of interference from professionals imposing an ill-fitting frame on the group, and the resources of the group, including the skills and abilities of leaders and members.

Internal factors have been considered in this chapter, such as governance, membership, goals, and social technology. An hypothesis is that the more extensively and frequently groups for a given problem communicate their experience to one another, testing and trying out ideas, the shorter will be the time to evolve a framework or adapt a template.

The external sociocultural or ecological context (Maton 1993) affects the process extensively. Often problems are staked out and claimed by a field of professional practice or by public agencies. This process by which new issues become crystallized as named problems and linked to public or private institutions is the social construction of social problems (Best 1989; Conrad and Schneider 1980). The sociology of knowledge about a problem in society refers to the views of the problem held by different groups and the ways in which these interests have staked out a claim to manage it. We cannot examine an issue without knowing the ways of thinking about or framing that problem that are available in that society at that time. What organizations, professions, or institutions had staked out interests in promoting their version of the problem? It is within this societal context that people initiate a new kind of self-help group that does not have a ready-made problem/resolution frame or a structure/process frame.[8]

The organizational aspects of the Caring Group as a self-help/mutual aid commons have been described in this chapter along with some comparisons with other self-help groups. This analysis details the development of a liberating meaning perspective, which is especially critical for short-term transformative (cell 3) and long-term transformative (cell 4) groups. Similar analyses are needed for other kinds of groups.

The general and, probably, universal social technology of self-help/mutual aid is the sharing circle: individuals with a common problem listen to and tell their stories of anguish, potential, and recovery and in the process are comforted, do not feel alone, and gain strength from helping one another. When the transformative groups, cells 3 and 4, have a liberating meaning perspective, they can refashion a more positive identity in the process of problem solving and create a network of friends and egalitarian peers.

Antze (1976) has recognized the importance of the teachings of various self-help groups and the way in which they are shaped to be an antidote to what the group perceives its problem to be; he analyzed Alcoholics Anonymous, Recovery, Inc. (for former mental patients), and Synanon (for drug addicts). Chapters 5 and 6 have described the teachings of the Caring Group on Stuttering, how they learned about themselves and identified social technologies in addition to the sharing circle that could be helpful in solving problems. Saying one's name in front of others, becoming friends and participating in social events, and having external goals that involved talking were particular aspects they found that they needed. Interestingly, I would never have categorized friendship and social events as social technology if it had not been for the distinctive history of the Caring Group. They were initially warned against friendships and social events, but over time realized that they needed them—as individuals and for the maintenance of the group. As more qualitative research is done on the meaning perspectives of various groups, we can identity what is universal to self-help/mutual aid, what is culturally specific, and what is specific to a particular problem (Gidron and Chesler 1994).

Chapter 7

Transforming Individual Perspectives

*And the good part about the group most of the time is
each person expresses what works for them or does not
work for them. They do not say "Do such and such." I
would get very turned off. It's that you accept or reject
the things that work for you.*

—woman in Caring Group on Stuttering

*[It] seemed like the people you were talking to knew—
either where you'd been or where you were at, or, if they
were past you, where you were going to.*

—member of Families of the Mentally Ill
(Medvene and Krauss 1985, 1)

THE QUOTE by the woman who stutters emphasizes that the sharing in the group focuses on what works and does not work for each person; participants have to choose which ideas and perspectives apply to them personally. The experiential knowledge of the group comes to be knowledge owned by an individual. The words of the family member from the Families of the Mentally Ill group illustrate that participants gain perspective and learn about future possibilities from listening to others.

The experiential-social learning process, initially described in chapter 2, is a useful way to explain and understand how individuals can be transformed within the context of the group.[1] The individual participant obtains ideas and perspectives from the group culture and engages in a process of experiential learning both inside the commons and outside in the whole of his life. If the participant continues his involvement with the group, the three stages of individual transformation from victim to survivor to thrivor/advocate can occur. The three stages are somewhat analogous to the developmental stages that a group undergoes described in chapter 6—fledgling, developed, and mature.

In this chapter, I assume that the self-help/mutual aid group in which the individual learns is a developed or mature one with experiential authority and an established meaning perspective. A reciprocal relationship develops between the commons as a collectivity and the individual participants who compose it. Together the individuals create, transmit, and apply the knowledge developed within the group. Seasoned members trust their knowledge, value their experiential understanding, and possess self-authority about it. At the same time, a developed group as a whole has an "idioculture," that is, its own distinctive subculture—values, beliefs, rituals, language, artifacts, and a body of experiential knowledge and shared understandings about the shared problem. The idioculture is greater than that of any member and different from any member's idiosyncratic personal experience (Forsyth 1990).

Insights from the Field of Adult Education

A broad conceptual framework from the field of adult education encompasses the process of experiential-social learning better than earlier metaphors drawn from group therapy or human services. Many assumptions and principles from the field of adult education illuminate the experiential-social learning of self-help/mutual aid in the commons. A basic assumption of many specialists in adult education is that adult learning is best achieved in dialogue. Jane Vella (1994) defines dialogue as "the word between us," from the Greek *dia*, which means "between," and *logos*, which means "word." "The approach to adult learning based on these principles holds that adults have enough life experience to be in dialogue with any teacher, about any subject, and will learn new knowledge or attitudes or skills best in relation to that life experience" (Vella 1994, 3).

Many works on adult education, however, assume that learning primarily occurs within a formal educational system with a teacher. The adult education specialist addresses the teacher about how to design a safe learning environment or how to do a "needs assessment" in such a way that the learner participates in naming what is to be learned (principle 10 below). Paradoxically, the field emphasizes learner-directed or self-directed learning but often discusses it in the context of a teacher in a formal setting assisting the learner-managed learning. The insights from adult education will be valuable in the analysis of self-help/mutual aid organizations when they are framed within a broad community context, not the narrow view that education only occurs within schools.[2]

Vella developed twelve principles of adult education on the basis of her work in community education settings around the world. Although she translates these principles into the formal educational situation in which a teacher designs, plans, and implements the "educational experience" for her learners rather than the self-directed setting of self-help/mutual aid, I have reworded each principle as if there were no formal class or teacher. The self-help/mutual aid group is the teacher and the member is often both a teacher and a learner. Further, I have reorganized her twelve principles under three headings: characteristics of the learning context, the content and process of learning, and the learner. The principles apply well to developed self-help/mutual aid groups.

The following are characteristics of the learning context:

1. Safe environment and process (includes efficacy—the belief that the experience will work for the learner)
2. Sound relationship between the teacher and the learner (implies egalitarian relationships; hierarchical ones deter dialogue)
3. Clear roles and role development
4. Teamwork—use small groups
5. Respect for the learner as the subject of his or her own learning

Characteristics of the content and process of learning include:

6. Praxis, or action with reflection or learning by doing
7. Ideas, feelings, and action covered
8. Attention to sequence of content and reinforcement
9. Immediacy of the learning (the usefulness of what is learned is apparent)

Finally, characteristics of the learner include:

10. Participates in naming what is to be learned
11. Engages in what he is learning (emotionally involved, committed)
12. Accountability—the learner judges the success of what he or she has learned

The context of the learning environment was described in the opening of chapter 1 as a sharing circle. Indeed, the characteristics of the learning environment in self-help/mutual aid are partially satisfied by the definition of the self-help/mutual aid commons: a voluntary group of peers sharing the same problem who meet to solve that problem in a safe setting they control (principles 1, 4, and 5). The peer prosumer relationship is a form of mutual help as participants both receive and give help to one another reciprocally as equals by virtue of sharing the same problem and experiences (principles 2 and 3).

Naturally, the meetings and other activities of a real-world group do not always satisfy the conditions described above as the ideal learning context. Typical and ordinary dysfunctions and problematic situations occur in many groups, and occasionally even in well-functioning groups, such as a domineering personality who tries to control interaction, lack of leadership to maintain an organized and orderly meeting process, failure to keep interaction focused on problem solving and support, cliques that exclude participants, disagreement on goals, projects, or procedures, anger and conflict among members spilling over into group interaction, or lack of cohesion that jeopardizes the safe atmosphere characteristic of self-help/mutual aid.

Some of these group dysfunctions have been captured and measured by studies of "group climate," which originate in theory and research on group therapy. Rudolph Moos and his colleagues (1993) have accumulated a body of knowledge about the climate of the group that has been applied to self-help/mutual aid organizations. They developed and applied a "group climate" scale with ten subdimensions: cohesion, leader support, expressiveness, independence, task orientation, self-discovery, anger and aggression, order and organization, leaders' control, and innovation. Studies applying the group climate scale to self-help/mutual aid groups have found significant differences in member satisfaction and ratings of group effectiveness depending on the group climate. A number of studies show that in groups ranked high in cohesion, members perceive that they receive more support, are less depressed, and report higher self-esteem than members of groups low in cohesion (see L. Kurtz 1997, 39–42).[3]

Central to the idea of the self-help/mutual aid commons is the voluntary nature of participation that implicitly means that the learning is self-managed and self-paced. Participants listen and engage in issues as they choose (principles 10, 11, and 12). Within this context seasoned members may suggest or influence an individual toward a line of thought or action. Sponsor, guide, or buddy roles may be available in the group, from which novices can receive personalized one-on-one assistance from a more experientially knowledgeable member. Members also learn from their friends and acquaintances during social activities or other interaction outside of group meetings.

The self-help/mutual aid literature written by researchers has deemphasized the extent to which the process involves the active engagement on the part of the attendee, but Riessman and Carroll (1995) (as well as this book) seek to correct that impression. Some self-help/mutual aid groups emphasize self-help more than others in their public statements. Possibly groups in which members tend to become dependent on others, such as those for the hard of hearing, emphasize self-help. In contrast, AA emphasizes "mutual help" or "Higher Power's Help" as an antidote to counteract the alcoholic's perceived tendency to be overly independent and self-reliant. AA literature, however, indicates that recovery hinges on self-help as well as mutual help with peer alcoholics and help from one's Higher Power.

The fact that so much of self-help/mutual aid is grounded in experiential-social learning (characteristics 6, 7, and 9) is another reason the participant has to be extensively engaged and committed. Half of the central social technology of self-help/mutual aid—the self-help—involves the primary experiences of a particular concrete individual. So many conditions for which self-help/mutual aid are formed, whether our own or those of people we care about—addictions, illnesses, chronic diseases, stigmatized social roles, or coping with death, divorce, or other life transitions—involve intense emotional, mental, and visceral reactions. Unlike many medical interventions in which the patient can be a passive compliant attendee with minimal responsibility for active engagement, the self-help process will not work if a person attends physically without much emotional and mental involvement. Even listening to others in a meeting can be done passively or actively, half-heartedly or wholly engaged.

The Cycle of Experiential-Social Learning

The cycle of experiential-social learning described here is adapted from ideas of experiential learning from John Dewey, David Kolb, David Johnson and Frank Johnson, and others, and from ideas of social learning described by Albert Bandura as discussed in chapter 2. I refer to the process as experiential-social learning because so much of it occurs within a self-help/mutual aid commons in which an individual self-helper has peers to learn from and with. There we encounter the apparent paradox of "self-help," which is the experiential learning of an individual, in combination with "mutual help," which is the social learning in very special circumstances with peers.

It is useful analytically to divide the experiential-social learning cycle into four phases, while recognizing that the phases may not be distinct in actual practice (see figure 7.1). This process applies both to individuals and to groups (groups will be described in chapter 8).

In the first phase, an individual gains new information or insight about the common problem. This may occur in a group meeting, by listening to or observing one's peers before or after a meeting, by reading, or from a talk given by a professional to the group. Experiential peers usually convey information by telling a story about some part of their experience. Observing one's peers can involve a process of social comparison in which the person sees someone with the same condition and gains strength and hope (if she can do it, then I

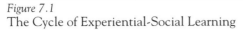

Figure 7.1
The Cycle of Experiential-Social Learning

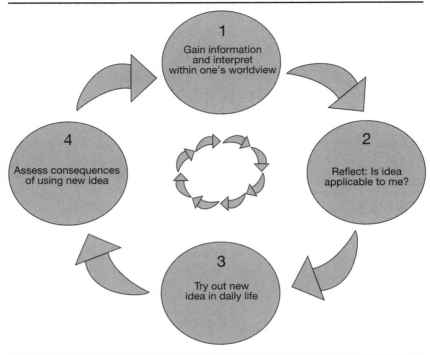

can do it). Downward as well as upward comparisons can occur (upon hearing someone's tale of woe I reflect to myself that I am better off than that person). What is relevant is that the individual gains some insight, perspective (way of interpreting a situation), or information. The commonality of experience of all participants increases the chances that individuals will identify with one another, which in turn means that they are likely to see similarities between themselves and others; simultaneously they also notice differences between themselves and others.

A number of observers emphasize that adults, with their established worldviews, have assumptions, often tacit or implicit, about cause-and-effect relationships, categories, and the meaning of concepts. Johnson and Johnson (1997) for example, describe adults with developed worldviews as having implicit "action theories" that include (often implicit) assumptions about cause-and-effect relationships. That is, when an individual observes someone and listens to his story, she interprets what she hears from within her personal worldview or "action theory." Nancy Dixon, whose formulation of collective learning is used in chapter 8 to understand how self-help/mutual aid groups learn collectively, refers to "meaning structures" as the set of assumptions individuals hold in their worldview.

Participants may identify themselves as similar to their peers or may fail to recognize similarities between themselves and peers in a specific situation in the self-help/mutual aid commons. In any particular situation one can select one's focus from hundreds or thousands of aspects of the other person, what she says or how she behaves or appears. Differences can be noticed and used as a means of distancing oneself from the others. So-called detached observers are assumed to be more objective and less biased in the positivistic-based methodological paradigm, but if the observer does not understand the frame of self-help/mutual aid group interaction, the conversation can be misinterpreted—distance does not bring understanding. Self-helpers' talk can sound like idle "small talk" because it is about the vagaries of everyday life, not the weighty issues of politics, economics, international affairs, or the equivalent.

The second phase of the experiential-social learning cycle is a reflective one in which the individual thinks about the applicability of the new information to his or her life. The willingness to reflect on the information depends on the person's engagement in the learning process; persons who do not want to solve their difficulties are less likely to engage in the reflective phase. The appeal of an idea to an individual depends upon many factors, such as worldview, values, current circumstances and resources, goals, priorities, and so forth. This reflective phase can be done alone or in conversation with others. Often conversations among self-helpers before, during, or after meetings, or on the telephone or over coffee contribute to such reflection.

An individual talks about the pros and cons of an idea in his own life or asks others about their experiences with the idea. Regardless of whether the individual tries out the new idea, the idea will be retained as part of the person's store of knowledge and awareness of how his experiential peers think, feel, and behave with respect to various aspects of the shared condition. This process generates recognition of diversity and difference from others as well as similarities.

In the third phase, the individual tries out the idea either as a change in perspective toward an issue or as a change of behavior. Individuals often go through this phase alone as an integral part of their daily life, but some self-help groups arrange for members to accompany one another in trying out new behaviors in public places (for example, groups for people with phobias).

The fourth phase is another one of reflection in which an experiential

assessment of the new idea or perspective is made. What were the consequences of trying this perspective or behavior? Was it useful to me or not?
Overall, did it work or not? This phase can also be conducted alone or with
others in the group. Often dialogue with others about one's experience with
the new idea gives the person perspective on what was useful or not as others
contribute to his or her assessment.

Meetings in which participants share their experiences are a forum for
members to compare themselves with their peers; part of this involves assessing the consequences of various attitudinal stances and behaviors. People hear
stories of participants with similar behaviors whose consequences were similar, showing them the connection between the behavior and its consequences.
The person sharing his or her story usually gets direct and indirect feedback
from others about how well he or she is doing. Laughter in meetings often
indicates that others recognize and empathize with the pattern; this feedback
is very rewarding for motivated learners and can lead to a change in perspective or behavior (Lofland 1969). An illustration of this critical learning process follows.

> When I come in there and I have this terrible story about how my
> speech just went to hell in x, y, z circumstances—other people relate
> to the circumstances. They ask me more about the situation and what
> was going on. They all agree they would be shot to hell, too, if that
> ever happened to them. I think, well, all right, then maybe it isn't all
> that bad. In effect, it cancels out the bad situation because I've said
> this happened, and they say well that ought to have happened,
> granted those circumstances, so you ought not to feel guilty that it
> happened, nor should you be afraid that it will happen again because
> now you know to do blah blah instead. And that might not have
> anything to do with the mechanics of making speech. (Dick, co-
> founder of Caring Group on Stuttering)

The four-phase process can be applied to this description. First Dick told
a story about an agonizing experience of stuttering in a specific situation. His
peers asked questions to make sure they understood the circumstances, and
they indicated that they would have reacted similarly in that situation. They
validated his primary experience. Their responses and suggestions for behaving differently in the situation came from their own experiential knowledge
of stuttering in such situations. Their reactions (phase 1: new information for
Dick) allowed Dick to question his assumptions about feeling guilty that he
stuttered so badly in that situation (phase 2: Dick had the insight that this
information applied to him). He also gained practical experientially based information about how to respond differently the next time he was in that par-

ticular situation. Dick also learned more about how his peers responded to that situation; if five members comment to him, he has new information from five peers who are both like him and unlike him (unique in their life stories).

The third phase, trying out the new insight or information in one's life, would be done outside the meeting whenever that particular situation arose. Would Dick react by stuttering as badly as he had previously? If so, would he feel as guilty about his severe stuttering? If the situation occurred frequently, such as getting angry at being treated disrespectfully in restaurants, then he could try out a different reaction within a few days. If the situation occurred infrequently, such as at Christmas or other yearly holidays, then he might have to wait months for the situation to recur in order to try out and assess a new approach (phases 3 and 4 of the cycle).

As noted, the cycle is experiential in that the new information is tried out or tested in one's own life. The individual's experience with the consequences of the testing (within the context of the group) is the basis for assessing its usefulness. The cycle is also social learning in the sense developed by Bandura in his social learning theory (1977, 1986, 1993, 1995). A mutual help group involves people pooling their information and knowledge about various aspects of the shared problem. They learn vicariously from one another, compare their progress with one another, and serve as role models for one another. Modeling or vicarious learning refers to learning from someone else's experience rather than directly from one's own primary experience. Participants point out the consequences of actions and reflect on the changes they see in one another. They set levels of expectations for themselves (don't feel guilty, Dick, when stuttering in that situation) and get constructive feedback about alternative ways to react.

This learning cycle facilitates the development of self-responsibility and self-efficacy, because each person arrives at his or her own decision about what ideas or insights to try or discard (Bandura 1977). Each person tests and assesses the consequences of the new ideas in his or her life (this is the self-help part of the process). Participants often ask peers in the group for suggestions or comments about what they are thinking or trying. In addition, some groups include mentor relationships: seasoned members help newcomers with these learning cycles. This reliance on peers is the mutual aid part of the process.

The experiential-social learning process becomes a more generalized mode of inquiry as well as a way to learn content about a topic. As a mode of inquiry, four features stand out. First, peers provide help in the form of reactions, suggestions, and positive and negative feedback, but they are not the authority or decision maker. The individual is the decision maker, which increases self-responsibility and self-authority (the conviction that what one thinks or does is valid for oneself, hence the development of experiential knowledge). Second, in contrast with our intellectualized society in which the capacity to verbalize is often equated with knowledge, experiential "knowing" is being or living something, not just the verbalization of something. The value placed on experiential knowledge is captured in the 12-step saying, "He can talk the talk but not walk the walk."

Third, experiential learning in a mutual help context becomes a generalized way of problem solving for some people. For example, I interviewed a woman whom I will refer to as Mary Lou who had belonged to Al-Anon, the 12 step group for families of alcoholics, for many years. When she had surgery for colon cancer and woke up in the hospital with an ostomy (an artificial opening in the abdomen for the elimination of bodily wastes), her first question was: do you have a support group to help me learn to deal with this ostomy? When told no such support groups existed in the hospital, Mary Lou telephoned the director and explained to him the importance and necessity of having a support group for cancer patients; with her advocacy efforts, a group was initiated. She knew the value of the self-help/mutual aid approach from coping with her husband's alcoholism through Al-Anon and wanted to reap similar benefits of information and support in coping with cancer and the ostomy. Furthermore, she learned self-advocacy in Al-Anon and could initiate a process that resulted in the creation of a support group in a new situation.

Fourth, self-help/mutual aid is inherently collaborative rather than individualistic. Self-helpers learn in the mutual aid context that others will and do help them, that successful problem solving involves working with others, and in turn, many self-helpers learn to reciprocate and help others; they become prosumers.

OBSERVING PEERS

Simply observing experiential peers for the first time can be a profound experience for newcomers who feel stigmatized by their condition and believe that people like themselves are "weird" or "abnormal." In chapter 5, in an initial meeting, Sally expressed relief at observing accomplished people who stuttered who were normal looking in appearance, and commented that they were not "oddballs or black sheep." Another example of the importance of visually observing peers is provided by a man who has been a member of AA and sober for ten years; he refers to "seeing" three times:

> What I found in AA that I did not get from any psychiatrist—and the thing that was most important to me about AA—was the feeling that I was not unique, and above and beyond anything the psychiatrist

ever told me—that I was really okay. I got this feeling of being okay in AA because all I had to do was *look around me* and *see* other people who looked pretty normal, who were functioning, who had done what I'd done, or even more. That more than anything else, made me feel okay, because I could *observe*.(Emphasis added.)

The knowledge and understanding gained by group members is largely expressed orally through stories and in participants' being and acting in the world. The importance of directly observing one's experiential peers is critical in many instances. Observing an experiential peer directly (primary experience) is much more credible and trustworthy than reading what an experiential peer has written or a professional has said (secondary experience), especially for newcomers. This is especially true for physical conditions that affect one's appearance. For example, some people who have surgery that creates an ostomy or ileostomy wake up from the surgery with a physical difference that can be interpreted as a deformity. They are fitted with an appliance worn on their abdomen underneath their clothes. Will the appliance show? Can they still wear jeans or tight-fitting clothes? Will their "physical differentness" be apparent to others? Will it affect their sexual desirability to their spouse or significant other? A woman with an ostomy who visited people who had just had surgery as part of her volunteering in the self-help group said,

When you go to the hospital, we are supposed to wear clothes that will reveal ourselves—nothing extremely tight, but something that would show that nothing is going to show and they are going to be able to do the same thing. When they can see that you're living, walking around, that they are not the only ones in the world that had it, it seems to reassure them. Well, if you can do it, then I can do it. It seems to give them a boost.

The importance of observing peers is a manifestation of vicarious learning (or learning from others' experiences) and role modeling; the most effective role models are those similar to us who are struggling realistically to cope with a situation (Bandura 1995). The power of self-help groups lies partly in the combination of primary experience and intensified vicarious learning and role modeling, since one can identify with and learn from peers who have undergone experiences similar to one's own. Vicarious learning is more effective if a person sees the other struggling to overcome his difficulties rather than making changes easily (Bandura 1977, 1986).

With the proliferation of on-line support groups, chat rooms, bulletin boards, and other electronic communication among self-helpers, the importance of observing and seeing has to be reassessed. How do people recognize their commonalities and identify with one another in the electronic media? Are the bonds among self-helpers as strong as in face-to-face groups? Preliminary research indicates that people can form strong attachments, self-disclose, and obtain emotional and social support from participating in computer-based support groups. However, the question of how the exchange of information via computer replaces direct observation of a person in a face-to-face group has not yet been addressed. Anecdotal accounts indicate that children and other people with physical deformities believe they are not automatically stigmatized and responded to in a negative and pitying or paternalistic manner in a computer-based support group in comparison with the treatment they encounter in an equivalent face-to-face group.[4]

LISTEN TO AND TELL STORIES: LEARN THE CULTURE AND GAIN A POSITIVE IDENTITY

The role of narratives or stories is central to learning a liberating meaning perspective and to transforming one's identify from a stigmatized "spoiled" identity with a hopeless future life story to a normal and flawed human being with a hopeful life story. Carole Cain and others (1991) have analyzed the way in which listening to the stories of others and telling one's story about one's past experiences within the context of the group's liberated meaning perspective can be transformative.

A newcomer needs to learn the meaning perspective of the commons and how a storyteller's personal story fits within it. Listening to the stories of seasoned members allows one to gain a sense of the general meaning perspective of the collective through the voice of a particular individual. Melvin Pollner and Jill Stein (1996) use the metaphor of a cartographer mapping the terrain to describe how the "voice of experience," the seasoned AA member, instructs the novice through stories in what the "social world" of the subculture of recovery is like, the characteristics of the people, the diversity and disagreements among them, the history of AA, the processes and trajectories or paths of recovery and its pitfalls, and practices. For example, seasoned members describe the learning process to newcomers by saying that when they first came in they did not understand the steps or they did not think they were alcoholics. Over time as they attended meetings and learned more, they began to understand the steps and they realized they were alcoholics.[5]

Simultaneously, while novices learn these and other aspects of the subculture of the group, they begin telling their story or parts of their story within the shared meaning perspective. This personal storytelling is an important way to begin reinterpreting one's past actions and history—one's identity. Within the context of the stories available to and expressed by the collective, one finds a different meaning to account for one's past actions. For example, reverting to your old stuttering self three months after completing a certain speech therapy is evidence not of your incompetence and inadequacy but the failure of the therapy.

An example of how telling and retelling stories within the peer context both facilitate one's reinterpretation of the situation and reveals a changed perspective about oneself comes from a social scientist who observed a halfway house for alcoholics that used the 12 steps and other principles of AA.

> Through listening to stories which residents told about themselves, it was sometimes possible to detect changes in their self-images. For instance, at one group counseling session, one resident expressed disappointment with himself because he "had given someone the power to get to him"—he had gotten angry at another resident who had been ranting at the morning meeting. Other residents who had witnessed the incident reassured him. They thought that he had been quite assertive; they had experienced similar feelings but only he had expressed them. On two subsequent occasions, I heard this individual recounting the same incident. Initially, he indicated he had been disappointed and upset; later, he realized that he had experienced and expressed his anger in a nondestructive manner; that is, he had not gotten drunk! (Barrows 1980, 6)

The resident began by being angry and upset. His peers validated his feelings of anger but in effect disagreed with his interpretation that he was playing the victim. They reinterpreted his behavior as assertive and appropriate for the situation. He repeats the story several times to his peers in informal interactions—engaging in a reflective process of reinterpreting the meaning of what happened—and he ends up interpreting his behavior in positive terms, finding that he had gotten angry but had not reacted by drinking alcohol and getting drunk.

The incident illustrates what many in the 12-step programs mean when they interpret so much of what happens in spiritual (but not religious) terms; spiritual as a way of being, in this instance, is an attempt to find positive learning results even in negative situations—the capacity to turn lemons into lemonade.

This incident also suggests the slow and repetitive nature of experiential-social learning to acquire a new role and changed identity. Unlike many aspects of the logico-scientific enterprise, such as the multiplication table, which can be learned once and retained with some use, learning a new role and personal identity with all the emotional as well as mental and physical connections can be slow and require many repetitions before one becomes comfortable. Behavior and identity change resulting from issues as multifaceted and complex as addictions requires a very long learning process through all facets of one's life. As described in chapter 2, Kaskutas, Marsh, and Kohn (1998) compare the way in which experiential learning is used in a self-help agency for recovering substance abusers based on the 12-step/12-tradition model of AA with an analogous hospital treatment program for substance abusers. Staff in the self-help agency are recovering alcoholics and drug addicts who use the AA approach; they help novices to see that they need to experientially learn how to work, play, celebrate holidays, relate to families and friends, and so forth sober and clean rather than inebriated or high. The program assumes that this takes months and years, not days or weeks as the hospital program provides. The program is oriented to facilitate their experiential learning in everyday living.[6]

The experiential learning process is complex, multifaceted, and nonlinear for both individuals and groups. If one looks at a single meeting, a cross-section of time, individual participants will be in different phases of learning about various issues. In a developed group one sees a range of longevity from the newcomer to the veteran. Even among people at the same stage, the salient concerns and issues for individuals will vary depending on their biography, worldview, values, current circumstances, and so forth. Furthermore, variation occurs because individuals learn at their own pace and troublesome aspects of the shared problem differ for each. As individuals participate over time, the four-phase cycle of experiential-social learning is repeated and repeated, and can result in changes of behavior or in some cases transformation of identity and lifestyle. The next section discusses the three stages of individual transformation that members can (but do not automatically) go through, changing their understanding and resolution of their problem and their identity in relation to it.

Stages of Individual Transformation

As individuals and groups repeat the cycle of experiential-social learning, they become more aware of what they know and are more confident that their experiential understandings are useful to them. Individuals and groups begin to take responsibility for changing their behavior and identity (regardless of what or who "caused" their problem). The accumulation of awareness, knowledge, and responsibility (changed behavior) occurs in different developmental stages. A three-stage process of individual development in experiential knowledge and identity change is posited here.

The stages of transformation described below are beyond "getting prepared" to change or making a commitment to change by affiliating and participating in a group—an initial step postulated by some researchers. Rather, I assume that people are attending a group and are involved in changing, and ask what kinds of changes in authority, sense of agency, and responsibility and identity they make. My developmental model cross-cuts other models in that it deals with stages of transformation in people who are making changes. The model considers issues of human agency, taking responsibility for one's actions, and change in identity from being a victim to a survivor—a model of empowerment.[7]

In table 7.1, the three-stage process of individual development is shown along with the characteristics of each stage. The victim, survivor, and thrivor stages of individual development are analogous to the learning stages through which craftspeople progress: the victim is analogous to an apprentice who needs a great deal of instruction and guidance; the survivor resembles a more seasoned journeyman who can work independently on routine issues; the individual at the third stage of certainty is like the master craftsman who handles specialized as well as routine aspects of the work and can instruct the apprentice and guide the journeyman.

In the first stage, that of the "victim," the person is apt to act like a victim—hurting from her raw experiences and unlikely to feel that her experience is useful. People come to the self-help group in pain, needy and vulnerable. They are usually "reactive" in their subjectivity in that they do not see themselves as the agents of their actions or link their actions to their consequences. In addition, depending on the disease or social condition they are experiencing, they may also have low self-esteem and self-hatred, be emotionally numb, or have a number of strong feelings such as despair, anger, shame, and vulnerability. They have a "spoiled" identity that can range in severity from bruised to rotten. They are the complainers and whiners that self-help bashers erroneously believe to be the whole of self-help/mutual aid.

The stage 1 victim in the Caring Group on Stuttering thinks that he is "weird" and often attributes any and all negative aspects of himself to his stuttering. Any failure of speech therapy is a personal failure, not the failure of the therapy, and so forth. Yoshida's (1998) concept of the "disabled identity as the total self" fits the stage 1 victim. I would argue that Yoshida's category of the "supernormal," the person with the disability who claims to be more normal than normal, is also in stage 1, because he or she is not realistic about the situation. As described in the story of the Caring Group on Stuttering, sometimes the mere observation of accomplished and normal-looking people in the group can very quickly begin to change the participant's ideas of what people like "us" are like.

The novice in stage 1 needs guidance from the seasoned members to learn and assimilate the meaning perspective of the group and to begin to retell his story in terms of that meaning perspective. A number of researchers have analyzed the kinds of help that newcomers to AA are given, showing that the suggestions are simple and are appropriate to the person's capacity when undergoing physiological withdrawal from alcohol.[8]

As people participate in the cycle of learning in the self-help group by attending meetings, listening to stories, talking to people outside of meetings, reading materials, and trying out different ideas about what has happened to them, their sense of uniqueness and isolation is reduced; they are understood and do not have to explain themselves.[9]

At some point, they are told by others or they begin to recognize that they are helping others as well as receiving help through their participation. No matter how painful their experience has been, it can help others—even struggling through the pain can give hope to another. Being helpful to others, rather than just the recipient of help, is a critical dynamic of mutual aid that builds confidence and self-esteem. It is also a hallmark of the new form of voluntarism that self-help/mutual aid is generating. The exchange of experiences, solace, and encouragement by peers forms a nurturing environment. In the mutual aid context, the newcomer in stage 1 may initially receive more than he or she gives, but the equation soon changes by stage 2 to a more balanced giving and receiving as individuals heal and reach out to others. They reap the benefits of the helper therapy principle described by Riessman.

The learning is not linear but more like a spiral. For example, consider the incident described by the social scientist observing the resident of a halfway house retelling his story about getting angry with a fellow resident. In terms of the stages of development, he began as a stage 1 victim—he reacted to the other resident. He did not perceive that he was an active agent who had control over his actions. In retelling his story within the context of peers who validated his feelings but not his interpretation of himself, he was able to reinterpret his actions by seeing that he was partially an active agent—he got angry but did not drink in reaction to his anger. By the conclusion of this incident he moved to a slightly different interpretation of what he was like or capable of being.

Members gradually accumulate experiential knowledge and trust that what they know from reinterpreting their past experience in the group is, in fact, knowledge. The second stage I call "survivor," similar to the practice of a number of groups whose members call themselves "survivors." For example, women who have gone through cancer treatment with the mutual aid of a support or self-help group label themselves "cancer survivors," and those who have worked through painful experiences of incest call themselves "incest survivors."[10] They

Table 7.1
Stages of Experiential Development for Individuals

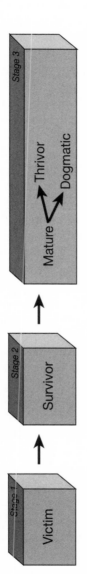

Characteristics of Each Stage

Identity	*Victim*	*Survivor*	*Mature*	
			THRIVOR	DOGMATIC
Use of personal experience	• Raw unreflected experience	• Confident of experiential knowledge	• Certain of core experiential knowledge	• Dogmatic about experiential know-how
Situation	• Hurting-wounded • Negative feelings (anger, despair)	• Healing stronger • Positive and negative feelings	• Strong and vulnerable • Growing/learning • Reframe negative experiences	• Strong • Stagnant/closed • Reframe negative experiences
Self-esteem	• Shattered	• Rebuilding	• High	• Moderate
Help status	• Needy, vulnerable	• Helps others; prosumer • Some needs	• Advocate, leader, guide • Recognizes needs	• Conditional help given; advocate • Recognizes needs
Subjectivity	• Reactive • Actions unconnected	• Self-determination • Takes responsibility for consequences of actions	• Self-mastery • Takes responsibility	• Self-mastery • Takes responsibility

have overcome their initial victim mentality and moved to a stronger place where they feel confident of their experiential knowledge, and have healed to some extent and recognize how their experience is helpful to others. By stage 2, the member has learned the meaning prospective of the group, and is adopting the more positive and hopeful identity that is available from it. The stage 2 survivor has come to view, in Yoshida's terms, that the "disability is a partial self."

A third stage of maturity occurs for some individuals. Individuals who continue to participate in the self-help group become certain about their experiential understanding over time and develop experiential authority. Many use their experiential authority to lead groups, become an advocate, or develop a career as a "professional experientialist." The professional experientialist is one who acts as a representative of recovered persons with that condition. He may serve as a representative to professionals or agencies that deal with his condition. Or he or she might obtain formal training and credentials and become a dual-status professional such as the ostomy nurse who has one herself, the recovering alcoholic who is a credentialed counselor in a substance abuse treatment program, and so forth. Such an individual may manage a self-help agency. Or, stage 3 mature self-helpers may become willing to lead self-help/mutual aid groups or help others in more substantial ways, such as serving as a sponsor or guide, or becoming an advocate for changing the victim's situation. A number of members of the Caring Group in chapter 5 showed stage 3 behavior—they became self-advocates for their rights to stutter in public, they assumed leadership roles like Dick to assist a national group to form, or they were courageous like Joe in admitting to people with whom he was developing relationships that he stuttered. Another illustration of a third-stage thrivor/advocate is Mary Lou, the woman from Al-Anon who advocated for a cancer support group from her hospital bed after having colon cancer surgery.

The stage 3 certainty can evolve in at least two directions: Some people grow and thrive, continuing to learn and change and becoming "elder statesmen" in AA's terminology, quiet leaders who are available to help but do not have to be in the spotlight. Others, however, become ossified. Their certainty about what they know from personal experience and participation in the group leads them to become opinionated and dogmatic. Some even become authoritarian: there is one right way to deal with the problem and they have the answer. Their identity is that of the orthodox. They are likely to help others conditionally, as long as the other accepts their authority and approach. They are called "bleeding deacons" and described as

> one just as surely convinced that the group cannot get along without
> him, who constantly connives for re-election to office, and who

continues to be consumed with self-pity. A few hemorrhage so badly that—drained of all AA spirit and principle—they get drunk. . . . Nearly every old-timer in our society has gone through this process in some degree. Happily, most of them survive and live to become elder statesmen. They become the real and permanent leadership of AA. Theirs is the quiet opinion, the sure knowledge and humble example that resolves a crisis. (Alcoholics Anonymous [1952] 1974, 139)

Passing through all three stages is not inevitable. A person can participate in a self-help group without going through three stages. They can stop at any stage. One can see people who have attended a group for several years who display the characteristics of stage 1, the victim mentality. Many people may attend long enough to enter stage 2, are comfortable with themselves and their survivor identity and discontinue participation, or participate at a stage 2 basis. Stage 3 people are those who go on to become leaders, special advocates, or "professional experientialists." From my observations, only a small proportion of participants are likely to continue to stage 3.

The stages of individual transformation model is useful for understanding what is going on in a self-help group. If I were to know one thing about self-helpers, I would want to know what stage of development of knowledge and identity they were in; then I could assess the likelihood they understand the meaning perspective of the collective or whether they were still learning it, their capacity to represent the culture and meaning perspective of the group and the extent to which they had worked through their personal problem. One of the biggest mistakes that observers, self-help bashers, and novices make is assuming that a participant in stage 1 with a victim mentality is a representative of the group and can faithfully represent its ideas, beliefs, and practices to them.

TRANSFORMATION

The self-help/mutual aid process can be transformative, especially in the types of groups that deal with persistently stigmatized conditions (the Caring Group on Stuttering represents a cell 3 short-term transformative group and AA represents a cell 4 long-term transformative group). A liberating meaning perspective is important in order for these types of groups to effect identity and lifestyle change. Transforming one's view of oneself from the stigmatized "spoiled" fruit to an unstigmatized ripe fruit with a small blemish (that is, the spirituality of imperfection in Kurtz and Ketcham's [1992] terms) is facilitated by the normal-smith midwife that the self-help/mutual aid support and liberating perspective provide.

Carole Cain's (1991) analysis of the way that self-helpers' identities are reflected in the way they tell their story of themselves is instructive. As pre-viously described, newcomers have to learn the group's meaning perspective, and as they listen to stories of stage 2 and 3 members, they learn that a new kind of identity is possible to have. But if they do not accept the new per-spective and modify their behaviors, they continue as they were. Cain first identified the major features of AA's "meaning perspective" and how stories of recovering alcoholics (those with a liberating meaning perspective) were constructed in the official literature as well as by members of current groups. Then she interviewed three newcomers, asking them to tell her about them-selves and their drinking problem. She compared the stories of these three individuals with the stage 2 and 3 stories of successfully recovering alcohol-ics. On the basis of what she had learned from the sober stories, she predicted which of the three newcomers would continue their AA participation and stay sober because of the story they told about themselves. Six months later she interviewed them again and obtained information about their current participation in AA and drinking status; her predictions were correct in all three cases. Although she had a very small sample, she showed that the liber-ating meaning perspective of AA can be translated into a coherent sense of how individuals' stories are framed and that there can be a correspondence between the story someone tells a researcher and his or her current identity and behavior.

Ellen, a long-term member of the Caring Group on Stuttering, described her five-month encounter with group therapy. Her story of group therapy is told here to illustrate her stage 3 transformed identity and empowered behav-ior. The group was composed of six to eight upper-middle-class normal "Beau-tiful People" (as she described them) and two psychologists. The therapists focused on her stuttering with the attitude that there was basically something "wrong" with someone who stutters. The male psychotherapist made, in her words, the "fatal mistake" of saying that she would be more attractive if she were fluent. She reports that she "fought back," attributing her capacity to assert herself to her participation and support from the Caring Group over several years. "Only I have the right to define the limits and responsibilities of my humanity . . . my ability to stand on my flat little feet and defend what I believed in was one of the most exhilarating moments of my life. I finally told him, 'if you don't like my stuttering, that is your problem'" (Ellen, the Caring Group).

Ellen is manifesting stage 3 transformed behavior. She has a positive iden-tity as a person who stutters and is empowered enough from her involvement in the Caring Group that she can defend herself. Her experiential authority about herself is strong enough to confront the socially legitimated power of the psychotherapists; she not only disagrees with their stigmatizing assessments of her as a person who stutters but also rejects their right to define her humanity. She was courageous to confront and disagree with the psychotherapists' definition of her situation. She felt "exhilarated" by defending herself in such a significant way (which indicates a great deal of personal empowerment). What a contrast with her stage 1 victim identity of self-loathing, perceiving herself as a "spoiled" human being, and reacting passively to the stigmatizing behavior of other people. Her stage 3 identity is not one of perfection but "ripe with a blemish"; she describes herself in a slightly deprecating manner as having "flat little feet"—in Yoshida's terms, disability as a partial self.

Ellen's portrayal of herself as empowered but imperfect fits with Kurtz and Ketcham's notion of the spirituality of imperfection that was described in chapter 2 (1992). Her claim that she has the right to define her humanity is a powerful statement; she shows the humanity and tragedy involved in the "community vision" that John McKnight contrasts with the "therapeutic vision" described in chapter 1.

SELF-DETERMINATION THROUGH RESPONSIBILITY

The stage 2 and 3 self-helpers learn to take responsibility for changing their identity and behavior, which is facilitated by the social technology of storytelling. Telling your story in "I" terms highlights how you view yourself: as passive reactor or active agent, as shown in Ellen's story. Taking responsibility for resolving one's problem leads to self-determination. Ellen showed self-determination in confronting the therapist and defining her own humanity.

An important part of taking responsibility is that by stage 2 or 3, the "objective" cause of one's problem in regard to one's personal situation becomes moot; individuals are solving problems for themselves. Simultaneously, they may believe that they did not "cause" their problem. Some may be motivated to engage in advocacy activities to attack systemic causes of their problem or barriers to getting help they need from the professional service system.

In a study of self-help organizations for African Americans, Harold Neighbors, Karin Elliott, and Larry Gant (1990) examined a variety of philosophies and manifestations of self-help in black communities in the United States. They found that even though the organizations were likely to view systemic causes as responsible for their economic and social plight, the self-help philosophy enabled them to separate the cause from the solution, and to work toward a resolution. The link between who is blamed for causing a problem and how it needs to be resolved is complex and not always logical from a scientific viewpoint. When the system is blamed for causing the problem and the solution is that the system needs to be changed, then the individual can be disempowered and feel helpless while waiting for the system to change (which is unlikely to occur in the short run). If the logical link that is typically held in science is severed between cause and solution, which it often is in self-help/mutual aid, then one can blame the system for causing the problem but still take responsibility for resolving it oneself.

Neighbors, Elliott, and Gant (1990) use the formulation of Philip Brickman and his associates (1982), who show that responsibility for cause and for solution are often not the same party, especially in social programs. Brickman and his associates looked at whether or not the individual is regarded as the cause of a problem and whether or not the individual is regarded as responsible for the solution. In distinguishing between the attribution of causing a problem as high or low and attribution of responsibility for a solution as high or low, they derive four general models that specify what form people's behavior will take when they try to help others (or themselves) and what form they expect the recipient's behavior to take. In the medical model, the self is not viewed as the cause and the self is not responsible for the solution either; the moral model is the other extreme—the self is regarded both as the cause of the problem and as responsible for solving the problem. In the enlightment model, the self is seen as causing the problem but is not expected to be responsible for resolving it; the compensatory model is the case in which the self is not viewed as the cause of the problem but is highly responsible for solving it.[11]

Neighbors, Elliott, and Gant (1990) pointed out that the successful black American groups followed the compensatory model. They argue that black Americans, the "victims," should and do pursue self-help efforts to improve their situation even though they are not the cause of them. The alternative, if they do not take responsibility for the solution, is that they will become disempowered, defeated, and despairing. Simultaneously, black self-help efforts should not let the government or society off the hook, since the system creates so much discrimination. In effect, a two-part strategy is used: self-help efforts are made in the here and now while advocacy tries to change the system in the long run.

SPIRITUALITY IN 12-STEP GROUPS

Behavioral and social scientists are predominantly secular and humanistic, but spirituality has recently become a topic of limited research. Aspects of spirituality are being captured in quantitative scales (an oxymoron?) and measured among convenience samples of AA members. Cancer journals also have considered how spirituality affects cancer patients (see Jenkins and Pargamet 1995). The recovery movement based on AA and other 12-step groups that has become a subculture in American life and the growing alternative medicine movement may have increased the appeal of the "spiritual" as a research topic (Room 1992).

The typical study examines a convenience sample of AA attendees (or substance abusers, many of whom have in the past or now attend AA). Some aspects of AA spirituality are measured. For example, Stephanie Carroll (1993) examined the extent to which step 11—prayer and meditation—and step 12—helping other alcoholics—were practiced; expressing meaning and a purpose in life were seen as an indicator of spirituality. Measures of length of sobriety, frequency of attendance at AA meetings, and other aspects of an alcoholic's affiliation with AA are ascertained. Some outcome measure, such as quality of life or having a purpose in one's life, is selected. These few studies consistently indicate that length and intensity of AA affiliation are positively related to sobriety and to a higher quality of life or having a purpose in one's life (Spalding and Metz 1997; Carroll 1993). In my terminology, the longer-term, more frequent attendees are more likely to be stage 2 and 3 survivors and thrivors.

Other studies show that length and intensity of AA affiliation are consistently related to having more friends, close friends, and non-substance-using friends, a finding that supports the idea that 12-step groups are types of self-help/mutual aid around which a community evolves (see Humphreys and Noke 1997; Humphreys, Mavis and Stoffelmayr 1994).

Despite the possibility of achieving stage 2 or 3 experiential authority, no research has been done to identify how many self-helpers in various kinds of groups reach these stages. In any case, experientially based knowledge is key to the learning process.

Advantages and Limitations of Experiential Knowledge

Professional observers and critics, especially behavioral and social scientists, often regard the experiential knowledge of the self-helper as anecdotal, implying that it is one person's biased opinion and that it is unrelated to any body of knowledge. Lee Kaskutas (1995) refers to this as the "N = 1" problem, that is, in research terms, the number of cases is one. She argues that self-helpers, in telling stories about their shared experiences, are each subjectively talking about one person's experience. "N = 1" does not apply to self-help/mutual aid in any simplistic way. The "N = 1" problem applies to the individual who reads a self-help book and tries to change his behavior by himself without discussing his issues with anyone—this is experiential knowledge based on one person's perceptions and behavior.

A new phenomenon emerges from the collective listening and telling, sharing, testing, and questioning of self-helpers inside their meetings and outside in their networks. It can be characterized as "disciplined subjective" knowledge or "collectively based experiential knowledge." However it is characterized, a developed self-help/mutual aid organization has a meaning perspective that has been forged from the anvil of experience of its participants over a period of time; the number of people involved in shaping it depends on the size of the group, its attendance, and its length of existence. (The evolution of one such meaning perspective was described for the Caring Group on Stuttering over a seventeen-year period in chapter 5 and analyzed in chapter 6.) As discussed earlier in this chapter, individuals learn facets of the group's perspective as they attend and listen, interpreting what they hear and see from their worldview. Individuals who maintain involvement will progress through stages of learning, knowledge acquisition, and transformation. The newcomer "victim" in stage 1 is more likely to be an "N of one," as newcomers are often self-absorbed and aware primarily of their own pain and travail. But the stage 2 survivor or stage 3 thrivor has listened to dozens if not hundreds of people over time. A stage 3 thrivor, a man who had been sober for twelve years in AA, described his experience: "If you come around AA, you have the benefit of being able to listen to hundreds of people rather than just one parrot . . . you have the experiences of a whole lot of people to draw on rather than the opinions of one."

Veteran members, after hearing and seeing many people share their experiences, come to recognize the finite number of ways an issue has been handled. They have learned about the variety and diversity of people's experiences with various aspects of the condition. A stage 2 survivor, a woman who had participated for several years in the Caring Group on Stuttering, put it this way: "As you are in the group longer, there are fewer things—everything has been experienced by someone else and you realize you aren't unique. That is one good thing about the group. You learn that—when you first come, you don't know."

A stage 2 or stage 3 member of a self-help/mutual aid group has a wider range of experiential knowledge, understanding, and wisdom than a stage 1 newcomer or a loner who has never problem-solved his condition with any knowledgeable peers. Neither the newcomer nor the loner would know the variety of ideas and feelings on various aspects of the condition, the various trajectories of problem solving and resolution, and so forth. In addition, the trap of dogmatism is less likely among those who have heard many people's stories of how to resolve the common problem.

ANALOGIES WITH CLINICAL PRACTICE

One way to understand the advantages for self-helpers working through their issues is to view their learning and problem solving as a form of practice within a collegial subculture. Often those critical of self-helpers or who misunderstand the nature of self-help/mutual aid are research scientists or others who hold different values than the practitioner. In showing similarities in practice between the self-helper and the clinical practitioner, as contrasted with the research scientist, new facets of self-help/mutual aid may be revealed.

The clinical practitioner often has to act to help his or her client on the basis of incomplete and uncertain knowledge. Self-helpers are in a similar situation: their level of discomfort and pain prompts them to act even though adequate and certain knowledge is not available. In contrast, the scientist is expected to suspend judgment and refrain from action until a predetermined level of evidence from adequately done research has been reached. Both the clinician and the self-helper are committed to values of health and wholeness rather than illness, whereas the values of the scientist are neutrality, skepticism, and caution (see Mumford 1983 for a comparison of clinical practice and medical research on which I draw).

Both self-helpers in their group and the clinician as a member of a professional network have major goals of helping reduce pain and suffering in the here and now. The clinician and the self-helper are interested in the whole person (although the clinician may define whole primarily in terms of biology or psychology). In contrast, the equivalent goal of the scientist is to demonstrate cause-and-effect relationships, to eliminate spurious factors, and to test and develop empirically verified theory in the long run. The self-helper, like the clinician, has an action orientation—seeking to try something to improve the situation. In contrast, the scientist is more cautious and takes time to design and conduct adequate research with a large number of cases over a period of time. The action orientation, combined with the urgency of the here and now situation, means that the self-helper and the clinician may take action before the theory is available to prove the benefits. Meanwhile, the scientist prudently waits to establish that a given treatment works as postulated by a theory. The clinician largely bases acceptable practice on what is commonly done by his professional peers; the self-helper in the group also relies on what he sees as customary among his experiential peers. The clinician and the self-helper recognize the importance of hope, and they hope that the intervention will work. The intensity of resolving meaningful real-life problems (which are life or death in some cases) experientially means that self-helpers and clinicians alike are likely to become emotionally attached to what has worked for them—their theory or approach. They can exhibit a zeal, passion, and commitment to their approach which is in striking contrast with the deliberately cool and skeptical demeanor of the scientist researcher.

These differing values and orientations help to make sense of the contrasting approaches of the practitioner (self-helper or clinical professional) on the one hand and the scientist researcher on the other hand. The limitations of experiential knowledge implicit in the practitioner's approach need to be acknowledged as well.

THE LIMITATIONS OF EXPERIENTIAL KNOWLEDGE

From the viewpoint of epidemiology, survey research, and other methodologies for studying representative samples in populations, the greatest limitations of self-helpers' experiential knowledge, like clinical practice, are that its conclusions are based on nonrandom samples and on the equivalent of only "treated" cases.

Clinicians and self-helpers tend to assume that what they know is common to the population, that is, that they have knowledge based on a representative sample of people like them. This is very unlikely. For example, the participants in the Caring Group on Stuttering are likely to assume that what they see and hear in the group is representative of people who stutter.

By definition, participants self-select into voluntary self-help/mutual aid groups, and those who sustain involvement are likely to be active problem solvers, not those who cope by denying or avoiding their problem. Those who attend are likely to select meetings close to home, which are typically demographically homogeneous because of residential and geographical clustering. Studies such as Vourakis (1989) and Kaskutas (1998) show that members choose meetings with members like themselves.

The issue of "treated" cases involves those attending the self-help group; self-helpers are unlikely to know people who changed through some means other than their self-help group experience, such as the alcoholics who stopped drinking through a church, another type of self-help group such as Rational Recovery or Women for Sobriety, or on their own. Other people feel they do not need to change—the person who stutters who is successful in media or academia.

Another issue stems from some practitioners' passionate commitment to a theory or problem-solving approach. Practitioners, whether self-helpers or clinicians, can become zealously attached to a theory or approach that they know to have worked for them or in their practice. They may exhibit no interest in alternatives or how well alternatives work. Some of this is clearly dogmatism, but is all of it? Some, I argue, is certainty about their experiential knowledge rather than dogmatism. Many observers believe that AA members are dogmatic or authoritarian; they seriously entertain the idea that AA is a cult. I am struck by the reverse: I observe tremendous diversity in AA both nationally and globally. As further evidence accumulates, the findings of diversity are strengthened. Zohar's and my analysis of AA as an organization suggests that it is a flexible, open, self-organizing learning organization (see chapter 8). Do observers, scientist researchers, and other critics see and hear passionate experiential certainty among stage 2 and 3 members and interpret this as dogmatism? We need to distinguish between the zealous confidence or certainty of open-minded stage 2 or 3 self-helper from the truly dogmatic.

In professional work, a formal education, years of schooling, degrees or certificates mark differences in proficiency. In social learning no such outward stages of development are recognized or conferred but they are nevertheless there. I have suggested three stages of development and transformation through which self-helpers grow. First, they enter the mentality of the victim. Second, they become the more responsible survivors who cope with their travails and gain confidence in their experiential knowledge. The third stage can fork into closed certainty and dogmatism or openness and growth. The transformation of the self-helper is usually heralded by an increase in responsibility and contribution to the social and civic life of the commons.

Chapter 8

Self-Organizing Groups: A Case Study of AA

In essentials—unity
In nonessentials—diversity
And charity toward all.

—CHURCH MEMBER

M~AX~ W~EBER~ conceptualized the reigning theory of the developmental fate of emergent organizations. In his view, augmented by others, small value-based emergent groups, usually with charismatic leaders, inevitably face a succession crisis (even charismatic leaders get old and die): who will next lead the organization? Further, as the organization grows and produces satisfactory outputs, the initial uncertainty created by insufficient or erratic resources becomes more problematic; workers want to focus on accomplishing the mission of the organization, not worrying about how to feed their children. The paucity of rules and procedures becomes limiting and constrains workers' capacity to accomplish projects instead of being liberating, as was initially the case when the organization was small enough to discuss and reach consensus on decisions. In Weber's story, the organization either changed, usually in the direction of bureaucracy, or died. Bureaucracy meant the development of a paid administration with rational-legal authority and the will to organize and operate on the basis of written rules and procedures, written files, specialization, and a division of labor.[1]

Indeed, Weber lives on not only in the halls of academe but in popular culture. The imagery of hierarchical bureaucracy is deep-seated in the collective psyche and culture. Years ago I watched my eight-year-old nephew and his male friends start an "organization" while at play. They set up a hierarchy with a leader at the top, assigned others to different positions that required specialized functions, and began writing down rules and procedures for who would communicate with whom, and how the work of the organization would proceed. I was fascinated and shocked. At the age of eight they understood the basic concept of bureaucracy well enough to create their own.

In new self-help groups I have seen people unthinkingly set up a hierarchical nonprofit organization with officers, board, and rules and regulations before consensus was reached about the mission of the group. No discussion was given to the appropriate structure; the idea of a hierarchical organization was a knee-jerk reaction. An understanding that supportive functions are facilitated by the circle of sharing was lacking. For example, an emergent group adopted a model for a voluntary health foundation to raise money for research and professional education for a rare heart condition that caused sudden death, but the participants were still wounded and grieving over the loss of their loved ones and couldn't respond to the goals. In the case of the Caring Group for people who stutter described in chapter 5, they wisely began with the circle of sharing. They then quickly surrounded the circle of sharing with a hierarchical nonprofit organizational structure, but the hierarchy was not taken too seriously and it was not used to dominate some members or develop an oligarchy that deflected the organizational goals to maintenance of their power.[2] In some situations, a bureaucracy is efficient and useful—especially when a standardized product is being produced in large quantities in an unchanging environment (Morgan 1997). Self-help/mutual aid "sharing circles" that evolve into multipurpose organizations or health foundations with educational, research, and fund-raising goals as well as support goals may benefit from a bureaucratic form of organization.

With the hierarchical bureaucracy (or its slight variations) so ubiquitous and deep-seated in our institutions and psyche, are there alternative models of organization that better fit the sharing circle? Or do new informally organized organizations with sharing circles remain so or mutate into hierarchical bureaucracies? How do groups and organizations adapt, learn, and change while preserving their core mission and identity over generations? How do groups adapt to new kinds of members (demographic differences, differences in problem definition), or modify their meaning perspective to keep up with the times? How do they react to changing resources such as more or fewer members or growth that necessitates more formal structures?

This chapter presents such an alternative that violates our deeply ingrained ways of thinking about the need for a hierarchical bureaucracy. Alcoholics Anonymous is examined as an unusual, nonhierarchical, fluid, and open form of organization that evolved from the bottom up over a period of years. AA began and developed as a decentralized network of groups that retained the circle of sharing as their core social technology. A culture of experientially based learning evolved that was protective of local groups while allowing the development of a national and international level of organization that could accommodate AA's increasing size and complexity. But the national-level organization is controlled by its local groups.

This chapter presents the 12-step/12-tradition model of Alcoholics Anonymous as an alternative organizational model. While preserving the "sharing circle" at the local level as well as its basic organizational identity over a sixty-three-year period (several generations past its founders), it has evolved with a self-organizing design that gives considerable autonomy to local units (thus encouraging diversity in members with different demographic profiles and worldviews). In the process AA has grown to over two million members in thousands of groups in one hundred countries (demonstrating its appeal and viability cross-culturally) with a national/international service organization. Over one hundred groups have imitated AA's 12-step/12-tradition organizational mode. Other organizational analysts have captured the distinctiveness of the Alcoholics Anonymous model by referring to it as a minimalist organization or as anarchist.[3]

A conceptual apparatus is needed to frame the open, fluid, and process-oriented form that became AA; the structural analysis that is used to explain bureaucracy is inadequate. The concept of self-organizing systems found in the organizational learning theory literature seems promising. Organizational learning, a segment of organizational theory, claims to explain and understand how organizations, rather than individuals, change. A loose collection of conceptualizations are becoming known as "organizational learning" theories; Peter Senge's The Fifth Discipline (1990) is probably the most popularly known, but many other organizational analysts have developed their own formulations. The work on self-organizing systems is selectively applied here.[4]

My work in applying organizational learning theories to self-help/mutual aid organizations relies extensively on a collaboration with Asaf Zohar, a specialist in organizational analysis; his knowledge and expertise has guided the framing of organizational learning in the work we have done to understand Alcoholics Anonymous as a national/international organization. The following draws on our collaborative work but any errors or oversimplications are mine.[5]

A careful reading of many formulations of organizational learning shows that models of individual cognitive functioning have been applied without modification to group-level learning. Individual cognitive functioning, however, cannot be automatically transferred to the group level. Groups and organizations, though composed of individual members, are emergent, in the sense that group-level facets emerge that are not traceable to any or all individual members. The name of the group, its technology for conducting meetings, or its social climate cannot be predicted, for example, from knowledge of an individual member. Accordingly, any formulation of how the group learns cannot be based on an individual model of learning. We found two exceptions in which the analytic unit was the group or organization, not an individual, and an appropriate formulation of how a group/organization learns was presented (Cook and Yanow 1993; Dixon 1994).

I will first use the insights of Scott Cook and Dvora Yanow to describe how local AA groups follow a process that creates a "culture of learning" which allows both for the preservation of core beliefs and values and for diversity in membership (demographically, ideologically, and in worldviews) and cross-culturally (in terms of values, beliefs, national welfare systems, and understandings). Nancy Dixon's model of collective learning will then be considered and applied to the "culture of learning" of local groups described in the first section. The last section of the chapter will briefly summarize the self-organizing metaphor. Its imagery will be applied to show how AA evolved its distinctive model of local group autonomy with the national-level organization as the handmaiden of local groups: an inverted pyramid.

The Culture of Collective Learning of a Local Group

Cook and Yanow (1993) applied their ideas of organizational learning to three flute factories in New England that were able to both preserve the quality and sound of their world-class flutes over several generations of workers and to change materials and adapt to environmental conditions. No one, two, or three craftsmen could have made a flute in any of the factories, but the combined and specialized skills of a number of mastercraftsmen were needed to construct the finished flute. The expertise and wisdom resided at the cultural level of each organization, not with any one individual. Culture was defined as shared meanings and understandings, artifacts, values, and practices, many of which were tacit. Cook and Yanow point out that the dynamic and ongoing preservation of organizational identity in a changing environment is as important to understand and study as the way in which organizations learn new lessons and unlearn outlived ones.

The concept of organizational culture has become a preferred way of describing the shared meanings and understandings, symbols and artifacts, and beliefs and practices that provide coherence and unity to an organization. This view sees groups and organizations as socially constructed realities that rest as much in the hearts and minds of members as in any written material (Morgan 1997). To clarify that each individual local group can be distinctive while being generally similar to other groups as part of a larger organizational culture, the concept of "idioculture" is used; it refers to the concrete and distinctive differences of the 212 South Main Street Sobriety Group in Podunk from the apparently similar Sobriety Group at 314 First Street in Podunk (Forsyth 1990); the South Main Street group has met continuously for twenty years and several old-timer alcoholics control the group, emphasizing the basics from the official literature; talk of illicit drug use is discouraged. Although the Sobriety Group uses the same readings and rituals in opening and closing the meeting as the South Main Street group, they have rotating leadership and are open to alcoholic/addicts' talking about alcohol or illicit drug use and recovery from them.

An international collaborative study of AA described in *Alcoholics Anonymous as a Mutual-Help Movement: A Study in Eight Societies* (Makela et al. 1996) shows that extensive diversity exists but that core beliefs and behaviors remain the same. Further, other ethnographic studies of AA groups in various locations are providing additional evidence of the simultaneous diversity and similarity.[6]

The central activity of a local AA group is its meetings. Two basic meeting methodologies are the sharing circle, in which all participants have the opportunity to tell their stories or parts of their stories relevant to a discussion topic, and the "lecture style," with a podium for the speaker and the audience in rows facing the speaker in which the speaker tells a longer version of his or her story, the so-called speaker's meeting.[7] The sharing circle is intimate and virtually all of the group have a chance to share and contribute to the dialogue.

The distinctiveness of the 12-tradition meeting technology and its importance has not been adequately described or understood until recently. Klaus Makela and his colleagues' examination of the AA meeting as a speech event is a good beginning to describe the distinctive technology and its significance that allow for the creation of a special kind of learning environment (Makela et al. 1996, chap. 11).

In all meetings, opening and closing rituals, such as reading a passage from official literature or saying a prayer, set the meeting apart from mundane ordinary interaction. Some observers describe this as the delineation of a "sacred space" in which conventional rules of interaction no longer obtain but new ones do; psychologists have described this as a "holding environment," a special place of interaction where members can work out issues and learn new ways of behaving in the safety of a sacred nonjudgmental space, following D. W. Winicott.[8] Special rules apply during the meeting, and participants behave differently in a meeting than otherwise.

Makela and his colleagues (1996, 140–141) describe ten primary rules of speaking in the meeting:

1. Do not interrupt the person speaking.
2. Speak about your own experiences.
3. Speak as honestly as you can.
4. Do not speak about other people's private affairs (that is, no gossiping).
5. Do not profess religious doctrines or lecture about scientific theories.
6. You may speak about your personal problems in applying the AA program but do not attempt to refute the program.
7. Do not openly confront or challenge previous turns of talk.
8. Do not give direct advice to other members of AA.
9. Do not present causal explanations of the behavior of other AA members.
10. Do not present psychological interpretations of the behavior of other AA members.

The first two rules are the most important. The first rule supports the distinctive nonconversational turn-taking system; the second rule restricts talking to self-stories. The nonconversational turn-taking system means that each speaker talks about what he or she wants, which may have nothing to do with what the previous speaker said. There is no "conversation" as it is conventionally understood. Observers debate whether or not the ensuing discussion can be understood to be dialogue, since people do not directly respond to one another's utterances. They may indirectly respond to a previous speaker, but it may be the third speaker before them, not the speaker who immediately preceded them.

This distinctive style of nonconversation can be confusing to novice listeners, and it may appear to them that there is no order, coherence, or development of ideas in a meeting. The talking can appear to be a jumble of unrelated individual opinions, ideas, and utterances, many of them couched in terms of the recovery language of AA. In fact, in many meetings ideas are elaborated and developed through the narratives of the participants that consider many facets of a concept like "trust" or "gratitude." One has to learn how to listen for the threads and commonalities that make up the "narrative community" underlying the meeting talk.[9]

The second rule of self-stories signifies the importance of personal experience and of relying on one's own or other members' experiences rather than expert knowledge from professionals (rules 5 and 10) or "revealed truth" from religion (rule 5). Talking is couched in "I" terms rather than "we" or general terms. Giving advice or lecturing is frowned upon (rules 8 and 9). The emphasis on interpreting the program for oneself and speaking in "I" terms is reiterated on the group and organizational levels. No one can speak for AA as an organization; no official spokespersons exist. The closest thing to a spokesperson for the entire organization is "conference approved literature," which refers to AA literature that has been officially approved through a policymaking body composed of regional representatives of local groups who meet annually.

The ban on cross-talk, that is, not allowing someone to directly reply to what someone else said, supports negative facework. Face refers to one's public self-image that every person wants to claim for him- or herself. "Positive face" refers to one's desire to be recognized and approved of by others; "negative face" refers to freedom of action and avoiding having one's actions impeded by others. Although the opening rituals of a meeting create a warm atmosphere and strong bond of politeness, unity, and solidarity, technically the rules of talk are geared toward negative politeness, thereby honoring one's need for autonomy rather than approval. "By protecting all participants against infringement of their negative face, AA rules of talk create space for derogatory and humiliating self-narratives that in other contexts would signify a total loss of face" (Makela et al. 1996, 143). Thus members tell their drunk-a-log stories of how they hurt and embarrassed others and themselves, displayed outrageous or obnoxious behavior while under the influence of alcohol, and got in trouble with employers, spouses, police or others, leading to their "hitting bottom." They describe their past and current errors, mistakes, and moral transgressions, usually within the context of the program philosophy and how they can apply the 12 steps or other aspects of the AA program to avoid repeating them. AA's steps 4 and 10 ask participants to examine and reflect upon their behavior and admit errors and moral transgressions as a preliminary phase to taking corrective action not to repeat such behavior.

The social context of a meeting is that of basically egalitarian peers who are attending to recover from alcoholism. The norms of discourse reinforce the egalitarian situation: individuals do not emphasize their income levels, occupations, social class, or other external characteristics that would serve to minimize identification with one another. Individuals share their personal experience in "I" terms within the context of negative "facework," that is, their autonomy and freedom to discuss what they want is ensured. They are not censured, praised, contradicted, or given advice; they simply give expression to their feelings about the discussion topic. When not sharing, individuals listen, often identifying aspects of their own behavior in what the speaker says about herself as well as facets of themselves that are different from the speaker. Members report that they learn to truly listen to other people and become empathetic to what they are suffering or otherwise experiencing. In this process participants who listen learn about the different interpretations that other participants have of some aspect of the program, for example, how they did the fourth step or what the idea of "humility" or "gratitude" means to them personally. Listeners learn a great deal about the diversity in people's reactions and behavior and how they approach and apply the program.

Novices soon learn to differentiate among speakers—who is a similar novice, who has some sobriety, who has a recovery program to be admired and even emulated? Seasoned participants listen differently to the newcomer. He or she is struggling to learn the seemingly esoteric language, steps, literature and other parts of the program from the old-timers who have years of experience working the 12 steps and applying the principles of the program to their everyday lives. How do members reveal their experiential knowledge and authority with the AA program or lack of it? Melvin Pollner and Jill Stein (1996) have studied how the "voice of experience" is conveyed in meetings: by reference to the number of years or months sober or involved in AA, by showing knowledge of the history of AA or familiarity with its official literature, by using the language, ideas, and ideology of AA, or by reference to service positions such as sponsor, program chair, treasurer, or representative to Intergroup.

The AA program is cast in terms of general principles (the 12 steps, 12 traditions, and the official literature) or the concrete stories of particular individuals. Each individual interprets the program or an aspect of it from within his or her worldview and understanding, which is related to such factors as: length of participation in AA, degree of involvement in working the steps, and having a sponsor. This diversity of interpretations and practices is further strengthened by a cross-fertilization of ideas that results from the AA practice of visitors from other geographical areas attending meetings. Especially in urban areas participants may attend several meetings a week, and thus the attendees at a given meeting are not a fixed and unchanging group. People hear different ideas at meetings depending on the composition of attendees (Messer 1994; Robertson 1988). Rural areas with few meetings or members, in contrast, are likely to become inbred, hearing the same few people's ideas and stories repeatedly. Evidence for the diversity in AA participation is accumulating, especially from Makela's international study of AA in eight societies: even among those committed to the program, "there are widely varying interpretations of what that implies," including different ideas about how important various steps are, whether they should be worked in order, done once or repeatedly, and how fast they should be worked:

> Part of the variability is related to the openness of the basic texts of
> AA. In addition, the Twelve Steps are learned and worked in

conjunction with other AA members. The oral tradition of AA
provides a continually changing context for working the Steps. AA
members also refer both to working "the" program and working "my"
program, it being accepted that "my" program may be different from
"yours." A survey of persons working 12 step programs in the United
States showed a wide range of responses when people were asked what
activities they had carried out in connection to each Step. (Makela et
al. 1996, 154)

On any given topic, the self-narratives that attendees share at a meeting
are likely to vary. Some pronouncements on a topic are contradictory if taken
at face value. For example, Jean will say she avoids having alcohol in her house
to minimize the potential temptation, but Ruth lives with her practicing alcoholic husband and finds alcohol all over the house. The listener soon learns
to put what individuals say in context, taking into account the speaker's living situation (living alone, living with practicing alcoholic, living with spouse
and children, and so on); but the listener is still left with extensive diversity
in the way that participants approach and apply the program. This diversity
in ideas and opinions means that ultimately the participant is forced to think
for himself. An anonymous member wrote in an AA (conference approved)
pamphlet "A Member's Eye View of Alcoholics Anonymous" that on any day
one can find an AA member who will in good faith agree with what the member has decided to do and can find an AA member who will disagree with
what she decided to do. "Thus, sooner or later, the recovering alcoholic in
AA is literally forced to think for himself. . . . The formless flexibility of AA's
principles as interpreted by their different adherents finally pushes our alcoholic into a stance where he must use only himself as a frame of reference for
his actions, and this in turn means he must be willing to accept the consequences of those actions" (Alcoholics Anonymous 1970, 21).

There are many indications that members are expected to make up their
own minds about how they work the AA program. For example, in the official literature, there are many references to suggested steps others have taken,
rather than prescriptions regarding what the reader must do. There are sayings such as: "Take what you like and leave the rest." The literature emphasizes that people come in with different beliefs and attitudes. If they continue
to participate and stay sober, they go through a process of change, some slowly,
others more quickly. An underlying and implicit premise of the AA program
is that it is self-paced, based on the individual's needs and situation rather
than a uniform timetable of when and how various aspects of the program
should be followed. Sponsors are more likely than others to make specific suggestions about what actions the individual should take, but if the participant

does not like the suggestion, he or she can ignore or "fire" the sponsor and sever the relationship (Messer 1994). Hence, while a sponsor or group may encourage a person to work certain steps or take certain actions, it is ultimately up to the individual to determine if, when, and how to proceed through the AA program.

A variety of opinions are held in AA meetings about all but a few issues. Important exceptions are that (1) abstinence from alcohol (or other mood-changing drugs) is the major prerequisite to recovery; (2) the alcoholic is powerless to control his drinking singlehandedly, but when he relinquishes control to a Higher Power, he gathers strength and courage to remain sober; (3) the alcoholic is not responsible for causing his condition; (4) alcoholism is a chronic progressive condition that is mental, spiritual, emotional, and physical in nature; and (5) if you want to recover from alcoholism, the AA program works if you get involved and work it. Even on the issue of abstaining from alcohol, however, if new attendees believe they are not powerless over alcohol and can control their drinking, members will say, you might need to do more research (meaning that you need to do more drinking before you decide you cannot stop drinking by yourself).

Newcomers are given simplified messages and regarded as vulnerable people who need to focus only on a few things, such as not drinking alcohol (or using psychotropic drugs) and coming to meetings to get support and learn the AA program.[10]

This account has described the skeleton of rules for speaking in a meeting as well as the narrative discourse in relation to the AA meaning perspective that allows local AA groups to create, re-create, and maintain an organizationwide culture that preserves the common and critical values, beliefs, and behaviors: abstinence, the 12 steps and 12 traditions, and principles in the literature and sayings and slogans. Simultaneously, this culture allows for the distinctiveness of its members' worldviews, behaviors, and sociodemographic characteristics. Local groups have extensive autonomy, a characteristic of the AA organization that enables individuals to determine the direction and character of their local group (Zohar and Borkman 1997). Many aspects of the practices, language, and rituals in group meetings as well as the interpretation of various aspects of the program are mutually negotiated and approved by a group's members. Consequently, the idioculture is a joint product of the group and its members, who typically have a distinctive mix of sociodemographic characteristics. Because this relatively autonomous process is repeated over thousands of groups with different profiles of members (worldviews, demographics, belief systems), extensive organizationwide diversity is found. In a single heterogeneous society like the United States, for example, there is extensive diversity. Once this dynamic process unfolds across national boundaries, even greater sources of diversity emerge in the different languages, cultures, religions, values, and welfare systems of the various countries in which AA exists.

THE CYCLE OF COLLECTIVE LEARNING OF THE GROUP

Nancy Dixon (1994) formulates a cycle of collective learning that does not reduce group learning to an individual's cognitive apparatus. She states that organizational learning involves principles different on the collective level from those involved in individual learning; however, she maintains that collective learning occurs within the context of the learning of involved individuals. Thus she considers the reciprocal relationship between the individual and the group.

In formulating her ideas, Dixon studied three organizations, two businesses (Chapparal Steel and Johnson Foods, both of which have profit-sharing plans for employees) and the World Health Organization. She looked at the World Health Organization (WHO) during its campaign to eradicate smallpox from the globe between 1966 and 1977. Although none of the organizations she studied was a member-benefit nonprofit organization, her formulation is especially pertinent to self-help/mutual aid commons since she assumes that all participants' ideas and actions in the organization are important for organizational learning.

Dixon proposes a four-step cycle of collective learning that is analogous to the four-step cycle of individual learning described in Chapter 7: (1) widespread generation of information; (2) integration of new/local information into the organizational context; (3) collective interpretation of information; and (4) having authority to take responsible action based on the interpreted meaning.

The application of these four steps to the WHO campaign will be briefly described to illustrate Dixon's work. In the first phase the widespread generation of information was accomplished through continuous data collection, especially by fieldworkers. Incidence of smallpox data was collected instead of politically popular information. In the second phase, new and local information was integrated into the organizational context by making data available to everyone. Negative findings were reported as well as positive ones, and headquarters staff spent one-third of their time in the field. In the third phase, the collective interpretation of data was accomplished by having everything open to questioning. There was a continual analysis of data, and when experience in the field so indicated, strategies were changed. For example, the initial strategy of mass vaccination was changed to surveillance and control. In the fourth phase, the authority to take action on the local level was given to fieldworkers. Policy decisions were made at headquarters, but fieldworkers adapted to local customs and brought local people into the decision making. The outcome was that several important changes in the definition of the problem were made and strategies were modified to conform with the results of experience. Dixon concludes that it was WHO's ability to learn that allowed it to continually make changes; smallpox was eradicated by 1977.

An individual's knowledge and assumptions about the world make up his "meaning structure," which Dixon defines as our assumptions and other ways of making sense of the world. These include our assumptions of cause-and-effect relationships, sequences of actions, categories to distinguish among things (for example, redheads, blonds, brunettes, and others), and seeing relationships in information: what is bigger and smaller or what is similar to something else. Tacit or unaware assumptions and information may make up 90 percent of our meaning structures. According to Dixon individuals receive sensory impressions of a subset of data and then interpret these impressions, which become part of our meaning structures; for example, Alice interprets Joan's behavior as shyness while Henry interprets the same behavior as aloofness—Alice and Henry are likely to react differently to Joan because of their meaning structures. Individuals have these unique constructions of the world because of their history, socialization, family of origin, and so forth, but they also share many commonalities with others from the same culture and society, and the commonalities are greater for gender, race and social class peers.

Dixon distinguishes the organizational members' meaning structures as private, accessible, or collective, determining to what extent individuals' meaning structures are privately held or accessible to others in the collective. Meanings that are held jointly with other organizational members are "collective meaning structures." An important point she makes is that "collective meaning" implies not identical meaning, but close enough accord that "members function as if they were in total agreement" (1994, 39). Dixon gives two propositions about the relationship of the type of meaning structure and organizational learning:

> 1. Organizations may vary considerably in the ratio of collective, accessible and private meaning. Organizations which have the greatest capacity for learning are those in which the accessible meaning is the most prominent, (Dixon 1994, 42)
> 2. Organizational learning is strengthened by making more of individuals' private meaning structures accessible so that they can influence other members, as well as by making the collective meaning structures accessible so that they can be tested and altered. In either situation the need is to make the meaning structures accessible to others so they can be exchanged and examined. (1994, 43)

Dixon's four-phase cycle of collective learning can be applied to the "culture of learning" that is characteristic of local AA groups as described in the previous section. The AA learning culture corresponds extensively to Dixon's conditions for organizational learning. Her cycle of organizational learning begins with the first phase of widespread generation of information, which she says is ideally collected from primary sources and includes the analysis of mistakes and successes. In the AA meetings most attendees speak from their personal experience, which constitutes a primary source, and a variety of information is generated as many people in the meeting speak.

Several aspects of the 12 steps are especially important for creating a nonpunitive climate for the examination of mistakes and successes. In the fourth step people look inwardly, making an inventory of their shortcomings, and then in the fifth step they admit them to another person (often their AA sponsor), thus making them semipublic or no longer solely private. The focus is on identifying one's own faults, not fault finding in the external environment (for example my wife, my boss, and so forth are not to blame for my problems). In step 10, people are encouraged to continually assess their behavior on a daily basis and when they do something wrong, to admit it and take corrective action. The attitudes found in these steps carry over into the ambiance of the meetings, which are safe nonpunitive places in which attendees can admit their mistakes and discuss possible corrective actions. These steps fit with Dixon's model, which emphasizes a nonpunitive attitude toward making mistakes.

The second phase of Dixon's organizational learning cycle is that there be a timely, frequent, complete, accurate, and unimpeded flow of information to the collective. Meetings of local AA groups are held at least weekly, allowing participants to share information frequently and in a timely matter. Being emotionally honest and not lying are highly regarded values for which members are positively sanctioned, especially when they admit mistakes or behaviors that are regarded as socially shameful. The admission of one's mistakes alongside the importance of being honest about oneself within the context of an examination of all parts of one's life means that much of an individual's private meaning structures are transformed into either accessible meaning structures or collective meaning structures. The group has access to much information about an individual's life and behavior that, in ordinary societal contexts, would be regarded as private. The group's climate is that it is okay to be vulnerable, to not have all the answers, to admit one's mistakes, and to be honest about one's feelings and actions, which is again a climate conducive to learning.

The third phase of organizational learning is to collectively interpret information. Dixon (1994, 79–84) proposes four conditions to support collective interpretation: (1) widely distributed information and expertise; (2) egalitarian values, especially of respect, equality, and freedom to speak openly without fear of punishment or coercion; (3) frequent interaction among subsystems, supported by mechanisms such as size and physical arrangement, and (4) processes and skills that facilitate organizational dialogue. The first and second conditions are met in AA by the fact that most people talk in meetings, and that the basic norms are egalitarian as already described. We have also seen earlier that the cross-fertilization of ideas takes place across meetings and geographic space. Meeting sizes tend to be between five and thirty people (Robertson 1988), which allows for extensive dialogue. The processes and skills that facilitate dialogue are found in the basic ten rules of discourse described above along with the fact that most members learn to tell their story to a group—many (even uneducated) members become very articulate in speaking before a group. Feedback is obtained indirectly, not by cross-talk at a meeting but by subsequent "sharings" of people who respond indirectly to erroneous information (L. Kurtz 1997) or by one-on-one sessions before or after meetings, over coffee or the telephone.

The fourth phase of collective learning identified by Dixon involves the group having the authority to take responsible action based on the interpreted meaning. Dixon states four conditions: local control, minimum critical specifications, no penalty for risk, and profit sharing. Zohar and Borkman (1997) show in their analysis that the control of the AA group is firmly rooted at the local level (tradition 4), and that AA demonstrates a commitment to the principle of minimum critical specifications in relation to the groups. For example, groups have the authority to take action, the autonomy to develop their own procedures and format, and the authority to determine their own leadership rotation. Indeed, any member of a group can request a "group conscience meeting," which is the equivalent of a business meeting to discuss and resolve group-level problems. The openness to the analysis of mistakes fits the condition of "no penalty for risk." Finally, the equivalent of profit sharing in a voluntary action context is that the benefits of effective group functioning are enjoyed by its participating members.

The atmosphere of not blaming other people (or by extension blaming other people in AA) but looking first at yourself and what can you do to shape up your own behavior is pervasive. If people can freely admit mistakes and aren't scapegoating others, but looking for their part in the trouble, then the situation is more conducive to a learning environment. In critical ways, the set of norms and expectations are "upside down" relative to those evident in "regular" society. If in regular society one does not admit to being frightened to lead a meeting, for example, in AA this is commonly expressed by the leader of a meeting, especially by newcomers who are not used to leading meetings.

This application of Dixon's model of collective learning has shown that the processes and procedures involved in local meetings are conducive to group-level learning. To what extent do the processes described above actually characterize the behavior of local groups? Clearly, the ideal has been portrayed and it does not fit all groups; evidence is available that groups develop their own quirks, dysfunctions, and idiocultural processes that deviate from this ideal. Many poorly functioning groups disband. No empirical research has been done.[11]

AA as a Self-Organizing Emergent Organization

One form of organizational learning theory draws on organic analogies. Self-organizing systems theory, based on metaphors from biology and chemistry, "suggests that complex natural systems adapt to change by mobilizing existing, inherent capacities to find novel solutions to complex problems" (Zohar and Borkman 1997, 532). Instead of the bureaucratic model of the centralized administration making policy, procedural, and other changes and imposing/disseminating them to local units, the self-organizing imagery posits an organization in which change emerges from the local units, in an organic, natural unfolding process rather than a deliberate rationally planned mode.[12]

This branch of learning theory considers how organizations can unfold from within dynamic internal processes rather than be deterministically designed from a top-down perspective.

> Contrary to our traditional understandings of successful organizing processes and forms, the metaphor of self-organization suggests that instead of trying to maximize centralized control and authority, it is possible to build on the strength of untapped, inner capacities for spontaneity and adaptiveness at lower organizational levels. It argues that social organizations may possess an inherent ability to re-organize and renew themselves in meaningful ways, without the need for central organizing bodies that oversee, direct and control change. (Zohar and Borkman 1997, 533)

Asaf Zohar and I examined AA in terms of the self-organizing learning theory literature. The self-organizing approach in AA can be usefully described as a series of organizing principles that avoids the traditional bureaucratic hierarchy, specialization, division of labor, and elaborated rules and procedures. The four principles are redundancy of function, minimum critical specifications, requisite variety, and learning to learn. AA emerged historically as a "context where organizational members are able to explore the *freedom to* organize in certain ways, as well as experiencing the *freedom from* the constraints of more traditional ways of organizing" (Zohar and Borkman 1997, 533).

The history of Alcoholics Anonymous shows that the liberating meaning perspective of the way to successful sobriety evolved in the first three years, coalescing by 1939, when the major text *Alcoholics Anonymous* was published. The process and procedures of operating local groups and the relationship of local groups to the national organization developed more slowly, especially between 1939 and 1954. The pattern set between the individual and local group was replicated between the local group and other organizational levels (district/regional and national levels): individuality and self-help is respected within a nurturing context of interdependence with the larger unit.

An analytical history of AA in terms of its organizational emergence shows that the cofounders Dr. Bob Smith of Akron, Ohio, and Bill Wilson of New York City discovered the major technology, the sharing circle of telling their personal stories of alcoholism and attempts to stay sober with each other in the spring of 1935. Bill Wilson, while on a business trip to Akron, looked for another drunk to talk to in order to quell a powerful urge to drink. Through a connection with the Oxford Group, an evangelical Christian group in Akron, he was led to Dr. Bob Smith, another "hopeless" alcoholic. When Bill told his story of drinking and hopelessness and his recent attempts to stay dry, the urge to drink dissipated for Bill. (Dr. Bob did not stop drinking for weeks.) The sharing circle importantly involved telling your story to a peer alcoholic and realizing that helping the other was beneficial to you (the helper therapy principle). Dr. Bob stopped drinking June 10, 1935, which became the founding date of AA. Bill returned to New York City after several months, and both cofounders searched for other alcoholics to help. Their initial efforts were unsuccessful; but after trying various approaches, they learned what worked to ensure their sobriety and to help actively drinking alcoholics who wanted to stop drinking. Both worked within the Oxford groups during the first three to four years, bringing the newly sober men to Oxford Group meetings. They applied ideas from the Oxford Group, accepting some spiritually based principles (for example, taking an inventory of your shortcomings and admitting them to another person) and rejecting others such as aggressive evangelism and their method of group control. From their experimentation they evolved the belief that unless alcoholics change and live a spiritual way of life, they cannot stay sober. The pragmatic emphasis on trying experientially to see what worked and did not work became a central learning process.

The Akron group had visitors who drove from Cleveland to attend the weekly meeting, but around 1939 the Cleveland group became an independent third group. Since members of the groups in New York, Akron, and Cleveland had different religious beliefs as well as other differences, the groups evolved different practices and beliefs, thus setting a precedent for local group autonomy. The geographical dispersion of groups also contributed to promoting mutual respect for group autonomy.

In 1938 members collaborated on producing the major text *Alcoholics Anonymous*. Bill Wilson wrote it, but all group members reviewed and vigorously debated the terminology as well as many other aspects of it until consensus was reached. The key idea of the "group conscience," or the will of the entire group based on careful deliberation, was born in this collaborative writing process as well as other cooperative actions during those early years. Democratic decision making is thus manifested in an AA group by the use of the "group conscience" to make decisions affecting the group.

Professionalizing AA in order to make money was considered by Bill Wilson but rejected by the "group conscience." A well-known, true, and precedent-setting story is told of Bill and others soliciting money from the millionaire philanthropist John D. Rockefeller, Jr., who turned them down, saying that, in effect, money would destroy AA. This became a turning point, evolving into a significant feature of AA: AA became a minimalist organization that needed little in the way of monetary resources, and what was needed was to be self-generated from the membership. Around the same time a national service organization, the Alcoholic Foundation, was established by the cofounders and groups as a tax-free charitable trust. It had five trustees, three of whom were nonalcoholic. The foundation was used as a place to publish the book *Alcoholics Anonymous* and until the 1950s was a platform for the cofounders, a service agency to the local AA groups, and disseminator of information to the public and professionals.

After publication of *Alcoholics Anonymous* (1939) and some favorable articles about AA in national weekly magazines, AA groups began to sprout up in United States and Canada in the 1940s. Most of the groups experimented with their own rules regarding membership selection criteria, procedures for conducting meetings, and group structures. Some groups flourished; others floundered or died. Many groups asked Bill, the cofounder in the New York foundation office, for specific assistance with group problems. Bill, following the pattern of giving suggestions to individual alcoholics, not orders, would tell groups about the experiences of other groups with procedures, rules, and formats. He shared experiences of the collective just as personal experiences were shared on the individual level.

The principles of group unity and the relationship among units—among local groups or between the local and national levels—evolved through a long, slow experiential process of trial and error, and by applying the principles from the 12 steps to the group level. The process illustrates the emergent organizing culture in AA.

Two critical phases of organizational-level development can be distinguished. First, the process of developing the 12 traditions that are the principles of group unity and the relationship between units and with the outside world involved information dissemination, thorough debate and deliberation, and democratic decision making among local groups. After much discussion, Bill was asked to formulate the collective wisdom into a set of key organizing principles for successful group functioning. He published a draft of the "12 traditions" in the organization's magazine, the *AA Grapevine*, in April 1946. Between then and 1950, when the 12 traditions were officially adopted at AA's First International Convention, Bill and other leaders visited groups around the country, and the principles were explained, discussed, reviewed, and finally accepted in an organizationwide learning process.

The second important organization-level process involved turning over the authority for policymaking and the direction of the national service agency (originally the Alcoholic Foundation, then renamed the General Service Board) to the "collective conscience of our whole Fellowship" (Alcoholics Anonymous 1994). Groups sent representatives to district- and region-level bodies that elected regional delegates. By 1954 the cofounders relinquished control to local groups through this district/regional structure and the yearly General Service Conference that held the ultimate authority over the actions of the nonprofit General Service Board. "Thus, an unincorporated body of group delegates who met annually at the General Service Conference was now the guardian of AA's core values and vision, and held the power to make policy about national and international-level activities, including directing activities of the General Service Board" (Zohar and Borkman 1997, 537).

DESIGN PRINCIPLES OF SELF-ORGANIZATION IN AA

The four design principles that have been found to characterize self-organizing units are redundancy of function, minimum critical specifications, requisite variety, and learning to learn.[13] That the last one, learning to learn, aplies to AA was shown in the first two sections of this chapter, which found that (a) local groups could be usefully viewed as idiocultures that preserve the AA values and principles while accommodating local members in all their distinctiveness, and (b) Dixon's model of how organizations learn as a collective fit well with the processes involved in local AA groups.

REDUNDANCY OF FUNCTIONS. Natural self-organizing systems have an excess of organizational capacity for performing a given function, but rationally planned bureaucratically inspired organizations tend to view excess capacity for performing a given function as inefficient or duplicative. The "redundancy of function" principle tries to build the capacity of the whole into separate organizational units or parts; leadership, financial acumen, and repair capacity, for example, would be found in all the units rather than in a centralized repair unit that serviced all units. In contrast, the rationally planned organizations tend to emphasize specialization, division of labor and an administration that is responsible for coordinating and directing the various parts and division of labor. Job enlargement is one small aspect of redundancy of function. Workers in a unit know one another's jobs and can interchange them; the idea is that when local units contain as many functions of the whole as possible, then they can decide how to change or perform various organizing functions in a manner that best suits their unique circumstances. The redundancy of functions approach is associated with bottom-level autonomy in order to allow local units to adapt to their particular situations. As described, the local AA groups have considerable autonomy. They have the freedom to interpret and adapt AA's core values and visions in diverse ways. Zohar and Borkman (1997) give examples of schisms among AA meetings on the issues of alcohol versus drug use or how spirituality is related to specific religious traditions or not. Makela and his associates (1996) provide much evidence of diversity in traditions, procedures, and rules of local groups across the eight societies they studied.

Above all, the operating procedures of most local groups are very simple, simple enough that a high proportion of participants can learn them; no rule book, procedure manual, or set of instructions is necessary. With AA's tradition of rotating leadership, a larger core of members are available who have practice in running meetings and operating the local group than in a typical hierarchical organization that may tend toward oligarchy. In the 12-step/12-tradition model, the core belief stemming from step 12, that serving the group as well as individual members helps your sobriety, means that a tradition of service to the group is encouraged by the norms and values.

Tables 8.1 and 8.2 summarize the organizing principles that AA avoids and those self-organizing principles of a learning organization that it has implicitly followed.

MINIMUM CRITICAL SPECIFICATIONS. Hierarchical bureaucracies control the lower levels of the organization from the top down. As a major mechanism of control, hierarchical organizations specify and elaborate what procedures will be

Table 8.1
Key Dimensions of Self-Organization in AA

Seeking to avoid an organizing culture that is—	Creates an organizing culture that is—
Deterministic, static	Open-ended, unfolding
"Top-down" hierarchically driven and controlled	A decentralized, participant-led, experiential learning organizing approach
Total dependence on the central unit for strategic direction and resources	Mutual dependence and support
Strive to streamline the nature of local diversity	Build on the energy, creativity, and self-organizing capacities of local groups
Mutual suspicion and mistrust	Mutual trust and affirmation

SOURCE: Adapted from Zohar and Borkman (1996).

followed and formulate rules and regulations that cover most eventualities. Written manuals, rule books, memos about procedures, and so forth are detailed, specific, complex, and thorough. Although these detailed and maximum specifications result in standardization and uniformity, they also inhibit adaptation to local situations and exigencies and thwart innovation.

The approach AA evolved is a striking example of the way in which minimum specifications can avoid the dangers of overcentralization while still maintaining a necessary degree of control and accountability over local group activity. Instead of establishing binding agreements that attempt to identify and prescribe every possible eventuality, a self-organizing approach aims to reach broad, shared understandings among different organizational levels. F. E. Emery and E. L. Trist (1965) described these as the "minimum critical specifications" that enable local groups to maintain their autonomy without compromising critical accountabilities to the organization as a whole. For example, the fourth tradition of AA states that

> With respect to its own affairs, each AA group should be responsible
> to no other authority than its own conscience. But when its plans
> concern the welfare of neighboring groups as well, those groups ought
> to be consulted. And no group, regional committee, or individual
> should ever take any action that might greatly affect AA as a whole
> without conferring with the trustees of the General Service Board. On
> such issues our common welfare is paramount. (Alcoholics Anony-
> mous 1994, S19)

Table 8.2
Contrasting Organizing Principles of Bureaucracies and AA

Bureaucratic *organizing principles* (*An organizing blueprint that produces* *structures and procedures that are* *"cast in stone"*)	*AA* *organizing principles* (*An organizing process and design* *that facilitates agreements that are* *"molded in clay"*)
Exhaustive specification of all foreseeable eventualities and contingencies	Reach broad agreements and shared understandings
Impose measures of restrictive control and accountability	Identify mutually acceptable *minimum critical specifications*
Maximize accountabilities, minimize local discretionary decision making	Minimize accountabilities, maximize local discretionary decision making
Centrally defined roles and responsibilities at the local group and organizationwide levels	Build in redundant functions at the local level: empower local nodes to determine roles and responsibilities on their own

SOURCE: Adapted from Zohar and Borkman (1996).

Local groups are unincorporated; their members organize and change their procedures following a general set of principles handed down orally by tradition or found in the official literature. No procedural manuals, rule books, or memos are available from district/regional or national levels of the organization to direct local groups. A local group may develop its own guidelines in written form for conducting its recovery-focused meetings and holding its "group conscience"–based (business-style) meetings, but they are strictly for the use of that group. Officially approved pamphlets on how groups can deal with external bodies (medical professionals, the courts, and so on), are available from district/regional or the national service body, but these are all described as "suggested" versus mandatory publications.

As described earlier in this chapter, the prototypical AA meeting as a speech event is organized as a loose structure that encourages individuals to talk about and reflect upon their own experiences and to listen to the experiences of others. It allows individuals to talk and tell their story (or part of their story) within the AA meaning perspective, using the organization's common language without restricting the content. Patterns of typical or acceptable content evolve in local groups, but they evolve informally within the understandings of the local people, which again reflects the autonomy and idiocultures of local groups.

Thus, with the culture of learning (described earlier in this chapter), local groups develop broad general understandings of how to conduct meetings and how to apply the principle of extensive local group autonomy and the 12 traditions to themselves. Participants attend multiple meetings in a local area and, when traveling, in other areas, in which they affirm similarities across meetings as well as differences (Messer 1994). The same approach of relying on a few general principles to guide organizational-level activities within a culture that is transmitted largely by oral tradition and by participants from local groups who are elected to be representatives to the district/regional and national levels ensures that the national/international level of organization is likely to replicate the approach of minimum specification of procedures and structures. Both the local groups and the organizational level of AA operate on the basis of shared understandings developed within the context of a few principles of individual recovery, group unity, and service.

REQUISITE VARIETY. The fourth principle of self-organizing designs is the idea that the organization will need to develop sufficient internal variety to effectively deal with its external environment. The insight of requisite variety was provided by W. R. Ashby (1960).

At the most basic level of initiating a local group, the requirements are very simple. Two or three alcoholics can start a group for sobriety as long as they abide by the 12 traditions and do not claim any other affiliation (such as belonging to a treatment agency). The ability of any two members to start an AA group allows extensive freedom to meet the needs of individuals and of changes in the environments.

It is on the level of local groups in a large metropolitan area that one sees the principle of requisite variety at work. In addition to general meetings for any AA member, specialized meetings evolve from the membership through their own needs: meetings with child-care arrangements, for gays and lesbians, atheists, young people, or nonsmokers. The evolution of nonsmoking meetings in the United States illustrates groups' responsiveness to changes in the environment. Until the 1960s or 1970s, in the United States at least, most meetings allowed smoking. The prevalence of smoking among alcoholics was high, as it was among the general adult population. Since the 1970s fewer recovering alcoholics smoke, just as there are fewer adults in general who smoke. In addition, during the 1980s insurance regulations began to prohibit smoking in community halls, churches, and other places where meetings were held. The combination of these environmental changes has resulted in more nonsmoking meetings than earlier.

One general principle regarding the spread of such specialized meetings was established by the governing body, the General Service Conference: groups for specialized populations cannot be exclusive but must be inclusive of any alcoholic. Of course the attendees are expected to follow the specific rules of that group. For example, smokers can attend a nonsmoking AA meeting; they are expected to abide by the special rule that there is no smoking in the meeting. A heterosexual alcoholic cannot be denied admittance to a meeting for gays and lesbians; older people frequently attend "young people's meetings." An exception to this rule is gender-specific meetings. Meetings for men do not have to allow females in their meetings, and women's meetings do not have to let men attend. However, these rules have been bent when a person of the wrong gender showed up who badly wanted to attend a meeting and no alternative meeting was available; the participants attending the meeting are likely to hold a "group conscience" session on the spot and decide whether to allow the person to attend or not.

Groups also vary in the kinds of meetings they host, their rituals surrounding meetings, and what other activities than meetings they host, depending on the needs of their members and local circumstances; other activities include celebrating AA anniversaries, taking meetings to institutions such as prisons, or having recreational events such as dances, baseball games, or ski trips.

Metropolitan areas or regional areas have a district/regional level of AA organization; intergroup agencies based on and governed by representatives from local groups and supported by the financial contributions of local groups act as clearinghouses that tell the public where AA meetings are, distribute and sell officially approved literature to groups, and have committees to work with the courts, jails, substance abuse treatment agencies, and other professionally based concerns in the metropolitan area or region. These units are organized more like a nonprofit organization, and they have identifiable officers, regular business meetings, committees, and written minutes of meetings, reports, and descriptions of agreements reached. They are organized in ways similar to professional and government agencies in order to be responsive to interactions with conventionally organized agencies.

AA's organizing approach exemplifies substantial organizational flexibility. The commitment to flexibility in AA is so pervasive that there are no provisions for punishing or dismantling "rebel" groups. The national service bodies have no formal mandate to sanction the activities of local groups. AA, in fact, is an organization that has no formal provisions for expelling members or barring groups from being affiliated with it. For example, the World Service Manual states,

It is probable that we AA's possess more and greater freedom than any fellowship in the world today. As we have already seen, we claim this as no virtue. We know that we personally have to choose conformity to AA's 12 Steps and 12 Traditions or else face dissolution and death, both as individuals and as groups."(Alcoholics Anonymous 1994, 73)

The tradition of allowing local groups considerable autonomy in shaping themselves is not seen as a threat to maintaining organization-level unity in AA; instead, it is repeatedly emphasized as one of its great strengths:

But this ultra-liberty is not so risky as it looks. In the end the innovators would have to adopt AA principles—at least some of them—in order to remain sober at all. If, on the other hand, they found something better than AA, or if they were able to improve on our methods, then in all probability we would adopt what they discovered for general use everywhere. This sort of liberty also prevents AA from becoming a frozen set of dogmatic principles that could not be changed even when obviously wrong. Healthy trial and error always have their day and places in AA. (Alcoholics Anonymous 1994, 105)

However, AA is deliberately inflexible in relation to efforts to change the 12 traditions and the 6 warranties (the last of the 12 concepts). The policy-making conference can, in fact, make changes to these organizing principles, but only after getting over 75 percent of registered AA groups worldwide to approve the changes. Furthermore, this all-group vote cannot take place prior to six months after its initial approval by the conference (Alcoholics Anonymous 1994). This procedure offers a rare glimpse into an aspect of AA's organizational and ideological foundations that is relatively immovable, given the monumental barrier of a worldwide, all-group 75 percent approval rate. Major system changes are possible but difficult.

It is apparent, therefore, that AA has adopted a flexible, fluid approach to the articulation of local-national relations. AA's organizational design is more a process that unfolds as part of a joint learning experience—molded as potter's clay, rather than cast in stone. It must be emphasized, therefore, that a self-organizing approach is primarily a way of thinking about design principles for decentralized organization rather than a specific structural form.

As we have seen, self-help groups, like other organizations, go through developmental stages. A significant part of organizational development is constructing and developing the group's meaning perspective as well as confidence and trust in the group's experiential knowledge. Groups that evolve to the third stage of maturity and have certainty about their meaning perspective are at a fork in the road. They can become open learning systems that continuously frame and reframe the degree of fit between their organizing process and design in a manner exemplified by AA as a whole. Alternatively, they can become closed and ossified, typified by dogmatism and rigid organization that imposes ideological orthodoxy on its members. AA has evolved organizationwide culture, principles, and processes that avoid "ossification." The significant level of autonomy enjoyed by individual groups, the upside-down pyramid structure, and the culture that positions the international/national level board and service organizations as "servants" to the local groups all are manifestations of this unique mode of organization.

The fact that on the local level, groups vary in their degree of openness or ossification is evidence that local autonomy is operating effectively to produce significant variety. Observers have noted that some groups develop oligarchies or ruling cliques of "bleeding deacons" who control the group for years; others develop oddball ideas at variance with the major AA culture or become cults with charismatic leaders who promulgate their own vision of sobriety and recovery (Maxwell 1984; Robertson 1988). Such deviations are to be expected if true local autonomy exists. With voluntary participation, participants do not attend meetings they find objectionable (except in rural areas or other situations where few alternative meetings are available). The social control of "deviant" groups is managed through the voluntary attendance; many groups that violate the traditions or ideology wither away from lack of attendees.

Implications

In summary, the AA's organization reflects its rich culture of experiential-social learning and collective decision making within autonomous local groups. Although this culture originally emerged in the course of developing and refining the recovery program, it has played a major role in shaping the way group- and organization-level modes of organization were formed. One of the visible consequences of this process is apparent in the emergence of the remarkably decentralized model of organization at AA that creates a context for successfully nurturing the emergence of multiple, diverse local groups around the world. Above all, the case of AA tells the story of a culturally embedded and culturally driven commitment to organizationwide learning. This culture of shared learning is ultimately rooted in the individually based experiential-social learning that takes place in the group meetings. The same spirit of shared learning is reflected throughout all levels of organization at AA.

Perhaps the most remarkable aspect of AA's organizing approach is the process by which it unfolded. None of this appears to have been deliberately set in place as part of some "master plan" by an organizing body at either national or international levels. Instead, AA evolved from the ground up over a period of many years: principles of individual recovery ("12 Steps" by 1939) led to the development of group unity ("12 Traditions" by the mid-1940s), which set the stage for the development of guidelines for organizational service ("12 Concepts" by the mid-1950s). Hence, while AA may exemplify the enactment of self-organizing principles, there is no evidence that these principles have been adopted in a deliberate, planned way. Instead, the present structure and organizing process that are evident in AA appear to have evolved and emerged incrementally over time, through a series of separate and perhaps isolated events throughout its history.

The emergence of these self-organizing design principles in AA are manifestations of an organizationwide culture of experiential learning. The pervasive influence of AA's culture of organizationwide learning has apparently created a context that has both nurtured and allowed some remarkable organizing forms and procedures to evolve. At both local and regional/national levels, AA has adopted a mode of organizing that is consistent with its grassroots, experiential approach to the recovery process. Historically, AA has been able to build upon the strengths and successful organizing experiences of local chapters, tap into local energy and creativity, and promote an optimal fit or congruence between the unique character of local groups and the organization as a whole. The organization has been able to avoid a traditional centralized bureaucracy, a rigid, top-down hierarchy, and strict measures of control.

AA's fluidity, flexibility, and responsiveness to participants, local circumstances, and situations undoubtedly interacts with attendees' experiential learning, growth in recovery, and stages of development and transformation. Obviously AA groups do not satisfy all attendees, since many attend for a while and then leave the group (Humphreys 1997), but among the participants who find some compatibility between their worldview and the meaning perspective of AA, the flexibility and autonomy of local groups means that participants are more likely to find a space for themselves to participate however they wish. Participants are listened to, they can contribute as little or as much as they want, and they are asked to pay attention to themselves and tell their own story within a meaning perspective that works for many people. This fluid, flexible structure allows participants to learn at their own pace, about their own issues, as they are able and willing; it increases their chances of learning and adapting the liberating meaning perspective to their worldview.

According to the literature, self-help/mutual aid organizations are thought to be protected from bureaucratic and oligarchic forces because of the self-help ethos that emphasizes participatory and democratic decision making. But the issue of whether or not groups enact self-organizing principles of organization is an empirical one. Little research has been done to identify the actual decision-making processes in local groups or the relationships and linkages between local and national organizations. Few studies of the nonprofit sector in particular have adopted theories of self-organization as part of a comprehensive empirical investigation. Research is needed on questions raised here, including: How do national self-help organizations evolve? How are they designed in terms of the self-organizing principles of design? How does a legally incorporated nonprofit organization (that requires a central board, staff and hierarchy) fare in practice with groups that have a democratic self-help ethos and that attempt to be collectivistic—that is, how can a democratic collectivistic culture operate in a hierarchical structure? Do 12-step/12-tradition groups that borrow AA's design and structure evolve a similar culture of learning in practice and exemplify self-organizing principles? Linda Kurtz (1997) contends that many AA imitators adopt the 12 steps but do not fully accept the 12 traditions as principles of group functioning, but research is lacking to substantiate that claim.

The self-organizing perspective from organizational learning theory allows one to make sense of successful decentralized, nonhierarchical forms of organizing such as AA. This perspective can help articulate a radically different understanding of the nature and basis for the successful organization of AA, characterized by the emergence of novel patterns at both the national and the group levels. It can help us understand why AA has flourished over the past sixty-odd years by building on the self-guided discovery of local groups who initiate creative alternatives in carrying out AA's values and vision. Finally, it can help us explain why AA has been able to coordinate a diverse array of local groups under a single organizing framework. In other words, it is precisely the absence of highly structured systemic rigidity and top-down, planned control in AA that widens the spectrum of organizing options and sets the stage for an organization to imaginatively seek new ways of self-renewal. Paradoxically, apparent instability and lack of control at the national organizational level become the source of the spontaneous initiation of new order or reorganization at the local group level.

The life-threatening nature and stigmatized character of alcoholism have affected and do affect AA's evolution and development as a voluntary association dependent on its members' willingness to participate. The life-threatening nature of alcoholism is credited by AA's founders and other observers with providing the motivation among participants that allow this minimalist and quasi-anarchistic organization to evolve. Desperate alcoholics founded and developed the organization in a last-resort context; they saw no alternative but insanity or death if they could not work together to maintain their sobriety. The committed who are desperate can set aside their bureaucratically embedded psyches to try an alternative group process; the uncommitted who might want to remake AA into a bureaucratic vision do not stay.

The stigmatized nature of alcoholism in the wider society acts as a barrier to people who might want to join the organization and manipulate it for their own purposes of power, social prestige, or self-aggrandizement. AA members joke that no one stays in AA by accident. The life-threatening nature and stigmatized character of alcoholism in contemporary society are supportive forces that facilitated its evolution and help to maintain the organization as it is, on the one hand, and are barriers to typical organizational pathologies of oligarchy, goal displacement, and goal deflection, on the other. Important and serious questions are raised by these understandings. With diseases, conditions, or situations that are not life-threatening or as stigmatized as alcoholism, can a model of an open learning organization such as the 12-step/12-tradition groups continue in a self-organizing manner or will it fall prey to self-aggrandizing participants, the dangers of oligarchy, goal displacement and deflection, and other sabotaging elements? Empirical research on other 12-step/12-tradition groups can help answer these questions.

Chapter 9   Conclusion

S ELF-HELP/MUTUAL AID has become an important kind of voluntary action that changes "victims" into helpers. It is a forum of adult learning, an introduction to the healing and transformative intimacy of the sharing circle, a service to more people with mental illness and substance abuse than the professionally based health and human services, an innovative social force that creates positive perspectives that destigmatize people with illness, social differentness, and disabilities, and an alternative family and community for many participants. It generates new creative self-organizing forms of organization. In addition to these "therapeutic benefits" are other social benefits that affect the community and the wider society. Through their participation some self-helpers learn the skills of public speaking, planning and organizing events, and how to administer other aspects of a voluntary organization. Social relationships of trust, collaboration, and reciprocity evolve between members and their support networks in the community as well as with professional providers, health and human service agencies, and policymakers in government. Some participants become self-advocates who can assert themselves to obtain appropriate professional services. They may also join with others in advocacy efforts to improve professional services, destigmatize their disability or condition, provide input into public policy, or make other social changes.

The number of people benefited by the various aspects of self-help/mutual aid is mostly unknown, as so many self-help/mutual aid organizations are small, semi-formal at most, and unnoticed by official statistics. Self-help/mutual aid groups constitute some of the dark matter of the nonprofit, voluntary and philanthropic action universe (Smith 1997a, b) in that they are undefined and not counted in official databases—along with other grass-roots organizations. The statistical reports of nonprofit, voluntary, and philanthropic organizations do not define informal and semi-formal self-help/mutual aid as part of the sector. If it is not defined and labeled, it does not exist.

The social benefits of self-help/mutual aid to communities and societies are even less known or appreciated because they have been all but ignored by researchers and observers. As described throughout the book and examined in depth in chapter 4, researchers and observers writing about self-help/mutual aid have framed it from within a "therapeutic vision," first as lay group psychotherapy, more recently as alternative human services. The psychologistic, that is, individualistic, approach emphasizes the benefits to participants but ignores the impact of the groups on families, communities, and societies because it is outside the typical research framework.

Taking a broader view—locating self-help/mutual aid as a commons (Lohmann 1992), that is, as one form of the third sector, which deals with nonprofit, voluntary, and philanthropic activity—will illuminate the phenomena more clearly, thoroughly, and expose hitherto neglected facets of self-help/mutual aid. By situating self-help/mutual aid in the commons, questions can be asked that are irrelevant from the viewpoint of the therapeutic vision. McKnight contrasts the "therapeutic vision" in the *Careless Community* (1995) with a "community vision." In the former, the good society is one in which professionally sanctioned therapy services are available to everyone. In the community vision that embraces self-help/mutual aid, ordinary people tell their stories of tragedy and triumph with passion and zeal in an inclusionary social space where people with warts and deformities have a role alongside the "beautiful people" (whose flaws are invisible) and the professionals are available to provide services but their viewpoint is not hegemonic.

"You alone can do it but you cannot do it alone" is an often-quoted saying in the literature on self-help and mutual aid. The phrase encompasses two ideas that are usually not joined: self-responsibility (you alone can do it, implying independence) and mutual aid (you cannot do it alone, implying dependence). Mutual aid refers to individuals joining together to assist one another either emotionally, socially, or materially; mutual aid can be neighbors helping a family rebuild a burned-out home or members of a self-help group listening to one another and providing emotional support.

Joining "you alone can do it" with "but you cannot do it alone" results in a "self-help group" or " self-help/mutual aid" and produces a special form of interdependence in which the individual accepts self-responsibility within a context of mutual aid—that is, giving help to others and receiving help from others. Individuals can maintain independence while they are receiving and helping one another. The whole of self-help/mutual aid is greater than the sum of its parts (self-help or mutual aid). The synergistic interdependence resulting from the combination of self-help and mutual aid is difficult for critics of self-help groups to see or understand; they seem to think only of a dualistic world where one is either independent or dependent.

Lohmann (1992) describes five characteristics of a commons, which he defines as a form of autonomous social action in which participants fashion their own worldview within the nonprofit and voluntary sector: voluntary participation, mutuality of purpose, member-owned repertory or shared resources, reciprocity in relationships, and relationships based on fairness, not law. The commons encompasses the widest array of social forms—groups, organizations, conferences, events, social movements, and advocacy groups—and thinking beyond the usual categorization of self-help groups as organizations reveals a wide array of diversity.

A Profusion of Flowers

Self-help/mutual aid is primarily a grass-roots effort that emerges informally, often spontaneously, by and for the people who share a focal concern. Professionals whose work involves the issue may assist in the formation of groups (Borman 1979; Katz 1961). Some self-help/mutual aid is initiated with the help of governmental or health and human service agencies such as the association for Alzheimer victims and their caregivers. A metaphor of self-help groups as wildflowers comes to mind. In a nurturing environment where there is water, they can bloom profusely, but they also often spring up in rugged terrain. Like flowers, self-help groups are living bodies growing organically and rooted in their environment. Some last a season and wither away; others survive to become perennials. Like wildflowers that come in many colors, shapes, and sizes, self-help/mutual aid is richly diverse in its organizational formats, social technology, relations to professionals, and perspectives. Wildflowers can be changed into docile domesticated flowers that the gardener tends and trims, just as support groups controlled by professionals and operating under the auspices of hospitals or other human service agencies can be docile and domesticated. But their wild cousins spring up unbidden along streams and roadsides; in fact, some self-help groups arise in reaction against their tame cousins in the professionally controlled garden. Many breast cancer groups, for example, arose in reaction to the restrictive rules imposed by physicians who took control of the earlier self-help group Reach to Recovery, Inc. And professionally controlled support groups sometimes evolve into independent self-help groups after the professional segment ends; or open-minded professionals begin with a plan to phase out their assistance after a group is established.

Three important distinctions need to be made amid all the diversity of self-help/mutual aid. First, 12-step/12-tradition anonymous groups like Alcoholics Anonymous need to be separated from the others. The others tend to be modeled on some version of a nonprofit agency with a board of elected officers and members, statement of purpose, and by-laws and constitution (or statement of governance)—the Caring Group on Stuttering fits this model. The organizational model of the 12-tradition groups is so distinctive that it needs to be treated separately from the nonprofit version (see chapter 8). Moreover, the 12-tradition groups do not engage in promotion or advocacy work. These organizational differences are profound, and we are just beginning to research them and their implications.

Second, a group's stage of development should be distinguished in terms of a meaning perspective and related experiential knowledge and authority. A three-stage model of development of an organization's meaning perspective and experiential authority was presented in chapter 6. The first stage is one in which fledgling groups struggle to develop their meaning perspective— how they define their problem, how they will resolve it, what is the social technology of the group involved in resolving the problem, and what is their new identity. In the second stage, a developed group has a meaning perspective that works for its members, and members have confidence in their experiential authority. The third stage is one of certainty of experiential authority; it can branch in two directions—toward an open learning organization or a closed dogmatic one.[1]

Third, it is important to recognize the way different meaning perspectives affect the changes that are believed necessary to resolve the problem and the length of time the member is expected to participate in order to receive its benefits. A typology was created with these two variables, following the work of Rosengren and Lefton (1969) done with formal agencies. Scope of change was dichotomized into small and extensive, and length of participation was dichotomized into short (about two years or less) and long (more than two years); the resulting cross-classification yielded four cells. Small change is labeled "coping," in which people are adapting to a situation but are not expected to have a personality change; transitions such as divorce, single parenthood, breastfeeding, and groups for significant others such as parents of children with cancer are major examples of coping groups. Extensive change is labeled "transformative," as it involves a change of lifestyle, personality, and identity; groups for addictions, life-threatening diseases, and many forms of permanent disabilities are prominent examples.

The typology of groups is useful for thinking about questions that include the different organizational issues each type faces and the kinds of relationships each has with professionals. As one example, the short-term groups, both coping and transformative, face the issue of generating motivation for members to volunteer to do the work to maintain the organization. It may be that professionally facilitated support groups are appropriate for many of the short-term coping situations. This new typology needs to be considered in future work in order to examine other issues.

Lessons Learned

I began writing this book with an understanding of the central importance of the common experiences that are the basis around which groups form and the fact that undergoing collaborative problem solving generates experiential knowledge and authority about their predicament. But the experiences that bring self-helpers together for healing and recovery are primarily negative— pain and discomfort, confusion and ambiguity, stigmatizing reactions from others, lack of empathy and misunderstanding from their support network, and often unsatisfying or inadequate aid from the professionally based agencies and organizations. The common experiences that draw participants together are inadequate to account for the transformative effect these gatherings can have on the identity and ways of living of committed members. Without the leavening effect of an alternative perspective that shows the potential of a constructive life-enhancing way of resolving the shared predicament, the process degenerates into the "culture of complaint" (Hughes 1993) or the whining and emotional exhibitionism on television and talk shows that we decry. The media excels in turning private anguish into a circus. Self-help bashers have confused the emotional exhibitionism in public with the problem-solving approach found in developed self-help/mutual aid organizations whose members' privacy is protected.

The group process by which a liberating meaning perspective is fashioned by sharing and reflecting, trial and error testing, and the spiral of experiential learning of a collective over a several-year period was described in chapter 5. The process was told in narrative form since storytelling is the major way that experientially based knowledge is transmitted and exhibited. Through an examination of the Caring Group on Stuttering over its seventeen-year history, the developmental process of fashioning a meaning perspective became transparent. The group began with a professionalized approach to stuttering that had been formulated by speech pathologists who were themselves recovered stutterers, normal-smiths who had a destigmatized approach to stuttering that was respectful, dignified, and effective. In effect, stuttering was redefined as a minor but incurable talking problem. Speech therapy could eliminate some extreme aspects of stuttering and help them become comfortable stuttering. Just as important, members needed, through the self-help/mutual aid process, to conquer their fear of talking (and stuttering) and come to appreciate that they were valued human beings with a slight impediment. Through this process, they came to own their own knowledge and authority about recovering from stigmatized stuttering, and their initial reliance on the ideas and authority of professional therapists diminished. They continued to respect some speech pathologists, but were wary of those who only claimed to know something about treating stuttering. Members were not antiprofessional, as the literature on self-help groups mistakenly labeled them; they were pro-experiential, exhibiting their knowledge which allowed them to challenge questionable professional practices and ideas. Because of this process of self-knowledge and self-authority, they became self-advocates—empowered to stand up for their right to speak in public, able to confront inappropriate or unhelpful professional behavior, and able to maintain their self-esteem and withstand stigmatizing interactions or other slights from an uncaring or ignorant public.

To understand how instant identification and bonding can occur among self-helpers, the insights of the psychologist Edward Reed (1996b) are useful. He distinguishes between primary experience—which we directly have through our senses of sight, sound, touch, and so forth—and secondary experience, which has been framed, selected, and prepackaged by someone else (that is, we hear something secondhand, read about it, or see it on television). Self-helpers' almost instant empathy, the intimacy and bonding that can and does develop, stems partly from the fact that they share a primary experience of the focal problem which has its own internal coherence. It becomes relatively easy to recognize when someone has undergone similar primary experiences.

A counterexample illustrates my point. I have observed and talked to women with lupus who attended a support group but could not identify with anyone because they did not have the same symptoms. Lupus is a disease that manifests itself in a wide array of symptoms: no two people may have the same symptoms (Maida et al. 1992). If people suffer in different ways because of varying symptoms, then phenomenologically they are not sharing a similar primary experience and would not be expected to instantly identify with one another.

The meaningfulness and coherence of primary experience explains why the bystander or observer cannot fully comprehend the experiential knowledge of another without having undergone it. I am often asked if the empathetic compassionate observer cannot understand the experiential situation and understandings of a self-helper (the person who stutters, the parents of a schizophrenic daughter, the person mending from open heart surgery). The answer is no. My experiential testing over and over again has convinced me that we can appreciate and understand some, but not all, of another's primary experiences. Equating the part with the whole is dangerous. A major reason self-help/mutual aid groups come into being is the commonality of primary experience; it is also a major reason for their efficacy.

Although observers have recognized that self-help/mutual aid is largely communicated through narratives or storytelling, the significance of this has escaped us. The humanities are expert in understanding narratives or stories; but to many of us in the human sciences, brought up on a diet of positivistically framed quantitative research, the not-so-subtle derogatory attitude of "they just tell stories" (the $N = 1$ problem) has infected us. Even slightly apologetic and defensive about our qualitative studies, we have not examined in depth what storytelling is and what it means. Storytelling can reveal assumptions and presumptions that are opaque in most forms of logico-scientific discourse (such as case records, research reports, statistics, and surveys). Storytelling is an efficient and effective way to reflect upon one's practice or craft, such as the craft of living that engages self-helpers. The assumptions underlying one's actions need to be examined and questioned in double-loop learning (Bateson 1972; Morgan 1986), and assumptions can be revealed by telling problem-focused stories. The liberating meaning perspective provides the framework within which stories can be assembled and ordered to reveal assumptions and meaning; the perspective focuses on the important versus minor facets and cause-and-effect relationships.

A related aspect of storytelling in self-help/mutual aid is that so much of its information, knowledge acquisition, and transmission is oral, not written—as well it should be, for knowledge is awareness that requires human consciousness, not digitally based information that can be stored in a library or a computer. Knowledge as "awareness" means that so much of self-help/mutual aid is "living," that is, embodied in the presence, behavior, and stories of self-helpers who participate in their group in the here and now. Unlike the member-benefit association that relies on its members' money and names for its educational or advocacy work, the self-help/mutual aid group relies on the selves (personalities) of the self-helpers to achieve its goals and to help maintain the organization. Self-help/mutual aid is a living and ever-changing commons.

Developing in the social container of the commons, voluntary participation is a vital characteristic of self-help/mutual aid and is also protective of other characteristics of the commons. When participants willingly attend, not because they were court-ordered to a group in order to avoid jail or prescribed a dose of self-help group by their physician or other professional provider, they can contribute to the continual renegotiation of the group's mutual purpose, they are more likely to reciprocate the help they receive by helping others, they will benefit from the common repertory or meaning perspective, and they will more likely be concerned with governance. If not, they are likely to be a negative presence in the meetings, attend intermittently, or drop out. A negative presence refers to an attendee who is physically present, usually because of coercion (having been court-ordered or the equivalent), but who does not want to be there, and who resists and rejects what is being said. In many states, judges are ordering arrestees with alcohol-related offenses to AA or jail; some AA meetings are swamped with court-ordered attendees (or busloads of detoxifying patients from treatment centers). With even a minority of 20–30 percent of negative presences, the climate of a meeting can change from problem solving to complaining. There are reports of seasoned members going underground and starting groups not listed in official AA directories to avoid such negative presences. Thus the health and vitality of the self-help/mutual aid commons depends on voluntary participation. Self-selection is a major aspect of self-help/mutual aid that the social science literature hints at but skirts around, perhaps not knowing how to think carefully about the issue. In emphasizing self-help, or the role of human agency and responsibility within the commons, the idea that extensive self-selection exists is a corollary. As studies have shown, only a small percentage of people (less than 18 percent) who are offered a self-help group and are told the benefits of participating will attend even one meeting. Greg Meissen and Mary Warren (1997) questioned leaders of self-help groups about how they would respond to an influx of members if managed care health programs prescribed attendance at a self-help group as part of their medical regimen; the self-helpers were enthusiastic about receiving more members. But I question how voluntary such attendance would be, because the patients have a contractual relationship with their physician and managed care health plan. Some patients might attend the self-help group reluctantly, as negative presences, in order not to jeopardize their relationship with their health care providers. At the same time, voluntary participation alone does not guarantee the vitality of the self-help/mutual aid commons. Many self-help groups wither away for a number of other reasons, including lack of members, internal organizational difficulties, or external barriers.

SELF-HELP/MUTUAL AID INNOVATIONS

A number of social innovations have been generated by contemporary self-help/mutual aid, including: (1) a social technology with both universal and particular elements—the particular ones designed as an antidote to counteract the problems that people with an illness, disability, or predicament have; (2) a new form of volunteering, created by the egalitarian reciprocal helping relationships formed in self-help groups; (3) a distinctive self-organizing learning organization, formed by AA and its offshoots, as an alternative to a hierarchical bureaucracy, and (4) self-help resource centers, which can be and are social incubators and "schools" for fledgling self-help groups.

(1) SOCIAL TECHNOLOGY. Self-help/mutual aid has developed a universal social technology as well as particular social techniques that are distinctive to a shared problem. The universal social technology is the sharing circle in which peers share primary experiences of the common predicament through narratives or storytelling; this intimacy generates and/or modifies the liberating meaning perspective through which the knowledge and learning of the group is transmitted and an individual can be transformed. The peer relationship is horizontal and generates mutual assistance and often reciprocity. The participant becomes a helper while receiving help (Riessman 1965, 1990b).

In addition, groups evolve other social technologies that help them find solutions for their predicament (as Antze [1976] importantly understood). For example, opportunities to speak in public found an important social technology for members of the Caring Group on Stuttering, who had to overcome their fear of talking (whereas that would be irrelevant to many diseases or conditions).

(2) A NEW FORM OF VOLUNTEERING. As a result of the basic social technology of the egalitarian sharing circle with storytelling, a new form of voluntarism is created in which helping others (being altruistic) is selfish and receiving help from others is altruistic (since you allow them to help you). This new form of voluntarism needs to be researched. In particular, we need to ask how self-selection into self-help groups relates to participation in other voluntary activities and volunteering in other organizations (see Smith [1994] for a review of studies of volunteering for the period from 1975 to 1992). We need to investigate to what extent this new mode of interdependence, rather than self-reliant individualism, becomes a generalized means of problem solving for self-helpers.

(3) A DECENTRALIZED FORM OF ORGANIZATION. Alcoholics Anonymous has evolved a decentralized form of organization that is open, fluid, and allows maxi-

mal diversity at the local level to adapt to changes. The 12-step/12-tradition anonymous groups have extensive autonomy at the local level operating within a culture and set of design principles (the 12 traditions). Local unincorporated groups control the national/international level of the organization through elected regional representatives who set policy at an annual conference.

(4) SOCIAL INCUBATORS. When I visited the Voluntary Action Centre located in the School of Business at York University in 1995, I was struck by the parallels between the Centre and the Self-Help Resource Centre of Metro Toronto. The Voluntary Action Centre was providing courses, workshops, certificates and degree requirements (training and educational services) for established nonprofit organizations and their managers. The Self-Help Resource Centre was assisting people with a problem who wanted to initiate a self-help group but who had no leadership or organizational skills to do so. New groups were formed and nurtured by the Resource Centre. Specialized one-on-one assistance was given as well as workshops, introductions to other leaders of self-help groups, written materials on how to start one, and so forth. The Resource Centre created a safe social space where newcomers could receive the help they needed to initiate and develop a self-help group at minimal or no cost; the language the Centre used, the informal relationships, and other aspects of its approach were appropriate to its participants. Ed Madara and his colleagues provide social incubators for new self-help groups in New Jersey and around the country; Ed reminds us that much of what newcomers need in trying to set up a group is "encouragement" and the positive models of successful groups. Other self-help resource centers are also social incubators and "schools" for fledgling self-help groups, although they are not formulated in those terms.

In the world of the marketplace, enterprise zones are incubators for small businesses where regular tax and other obligations are loosened in order to facilitate the development of economic enterprises. The self-help resource center or clearinghouse often assumes the role of a local social incubator but it is not recognized as such. Our society today does not value the importance of having a resource center that can protect, nurture, and facilitate the evolution of new self-help/mutual aid commons. For example, state governments including California and New York funded some self-help resource centers in the 1980s, but they withdrew their funding in the economic downturn of the early 1990s.

PROBABLE SOCIAL BENEFITS
Little attention has been paid to the benefits to community and society that self-help/mutual aid yields. The therapeutic vision has held sway in the

research on self-help/mutual aid, so we focus on benefits to individual participants. We lack basic information about how many participants in which kinds of groups have what kinds of friendships, mutual aid relationships, or other social benefits that strengthen the community. How many participants develop public speaking skills and other skills for running voluntary associations? Do these translate into participation in other voluntary associations that contribute to the democratic process? How do self-help groups contribute to a more caring civil society (Borkman and Parisi 1995)? What kinds of social capital are created? What kinds of social changes have been made because of these groups?

Recent research suggests the kinds of analyses that need to be made in the future. Keith Humphreys (1997), for example, considered the reduced health-care costs of sober alcoholics and concluded that AA, with its one million U.S. members, was providing a substantial if unrecognized service to society. John Messer and I (1996) asked how self-help groups contribute to social capital, using James Coleman's definition. Social capital involves social relations among individuals, aspects of social structure and organization that facilitate productive action that are embedded in relationships of trust, systems of mutual obligations, and normative systems with effective sanctions (Coleman 1990, 304). Following James S. Coleman,

> Social capital is defined by its function. It is not a single entity, but a variety of different entities having two characteristics in common: They all consist of some aspect of a social structure, and they facilitate certain actions of individuals *who are within the structure*. Like other forms of capital, social capital is productive, making possible the achievement of certain ends that would not be attainable in its absence. . . . Unlike other forms of capital, social capital inheres in the structure of relations between and among persons. It is lodged neither in individuals nor in physical implements of production. (1990, 302)

Messer and I conducted an exploratory study on the contributions of recovering AA members to social capital. We interviewed thirty members of AA or the family group Al-Anon from Los Angeles and San Francisco, rural Pennsylvania, and metropolitan Washington, D.C. When actively addicted and before participating in self-help/mutual aid, self-helpers were untrustworthy and unreliable in all of their relationships; sobriety and recovery had reversed those breakdowns and they had become trustworthy, trusting, and reliable with substantial improvements in their relationships at work, with their family, and in the community. Among other findings, we concluded that the self-help groups assisted in the development of the prerequisites of social capital, namely, individuals' capability to participate in trustworthy and reliable relationships. Coleman's analysis assumed that individuals had the capacities to contribute to social capital, but our research indicated that was an empirical question.

These and other issues concerning the contributions that self-help/mutual aid makes to the community and society need to be considered in research. A note of caution. Self-help/mutual aid is not a substitute for professional services, or a means for governments to abdicate their responsibilities to the poor and disadvantaged members of society. Self-help/mutual aid is instead a supplement or a complement to family, friendship, and other support networks on the one hand and to professional services and government responsibilities on the other hand. Barry Checkoway, Mark Chesler, and Stephen Blum (1990), among others (Riessman and Carroll 1995, Powell 1994), argue strongly that self-help/mutual aid should not be manipulated by conservative forces seeking to cut government expenditures in health and social services. The disadvantaged have lacked the minimal resources that have allowed the middle class to disproportionately participate in self-help/mutual aid in the commons. The professional and government sectors have a responsibility to assist the poor, racial, and ethnic minorities and other disadvantaged groups with resources that will allow them to participate in the self-help/mutual aid commons.

The Institutionalization of Self-Help/Mutual Aid

Institutionalization is the process by which a behavior, relationship, mode of organizing, or social process becomes accepted as the legitimate way of doing things in a group, community, or society. Institutionalization has a taken-for-granted quality; it is part of the culture that young people absorb like air without conscious instruction. Self-help/mutual aid is becoming institutionalized as an acceptable strategy of developing support, especially the 12-step/12-tradition form that Alcoholics Anonymous originated, and that has now evolved into a subculture of recovery (see Room's [1992] analysis of the subculture of recovery and chapter 1, note 6).

I told the story of my nephew who at the age of eight years made up a mini-bureaucracy with his friends while at play. This is an illustration of the fact that bureaucratic principles are so well institutionalized that young people learn them seemingly by osmosis. Will my grandnephew create a self-help/mutual aid group in play when he is age eight at the millennium? His father knew how to build a mini-bureaucracy at that age in the early 1970s. What will the next generation know? Is self-help/mutual aid that well institutionalized? If he creates one, will it be a 12-step anonymous group? If so, will he build in the "minimalist" self-organizing characteristics with decisions by consensus, rotating leadership, and deemphasis of social class, prestige symbols, income, and other divisive social indicators? Will the likelihood of his building a self-help group depend on the gender of his playmates? Will a group with females be more likely to think of self-help/mutual aid than an all-male group?

More and more professionals appropriate the 12 steps and fashion them into money-making propositions, which are at total odds with the original intent. The substance abuse treatment industry was developed in the 1970s partly through the entrepreneurial efforts of recovering alcoholics in AA who acted in their capacity as citizens, not as AA members. Ironically, a substantial part of the substance abuse treatment industry has appropriated the 12 steps and other ideas from AA and makes money from them. Critics fail to separate the marketplace from the voluntary sector, often attributing to AA or the self-help groups the activities of the marketplace, not the voluntary sector.

The epitome of the appropriation of 12-step ideas occurs when academic management gurus who consult for Fortune 500 companies or their equivalent adopt the 12 steps of AA for a spiritually based approach to management. Ian Mitroff, management professor at the University of Southern California, in *Smart Thinking for Crazy Times* (1998), proposes ethically based management that incorporates aesthetics, existential needs, and spirituality. In his interpretation, "the definition of spirituality in this context is one of the primary purposes of the Twelve Steps of AA. Thus, the Twelve Steps can be construed as a management process for defining spirituality, but only within the total context of an individual's or an organization's life and the process of giving new and revitalized meaning to that life" (1998, 151). Interestingly, he defines being spiritual as being continually open-minded and examining one's mistakes and errors to see what one can learn: spirituality as open-minded, but ethically framed, learning.

Ritzer, in *The McDonaldization of Society* (1993), argues that bureaucratic principles are being extended to more and more life areas through the processes of rationalization and bureaucratization. Ritzer's analysis reveals the underlying principles at work—efficiency, calculability, predictability, and control. He also describes small but definite countervailing trends—the bed and breakfasts, gourmet ice cream, specialty book shops, and so forth. Self-help/mutual aid is an example of a countervailing trend to McDonaldization. People participate as whole human beings, not in segmented roles, and the basic social technology is made up of sharing circles in which people listen to and tell stories of their pain and anguish, the potential and occurrence of healing and recovery. The experiential learning from this intimacy can become transformative. In problem-solving groups without negative presences, interactions are authentic, caring, and nonjudgmental; helping relationships and friendships evolve. In considering self-help/mutual aid in the commons, we are able to discover much more than the therapeutic benefits of its major process, which I call the sharing circle. In exploring underlying principles not previously considered, this book seeks to generate research on the newly asked questions.

Notes

Chapter 1   *What Is Self-Help/Mutual Aid?*

1. Technology is defined here in a generic sense as the means or techniques used to solve or resolve problems; social technology will refer to relationships among people and organizations, such as the "sharing circle" used to communicate personal experiences regarding the focal problem of the group. Technology is discussed further in Chapter 6.

    John Lofland is a sociologist who formulated a version of the societal reaction/labeling approach to social deviance in his book *Deviance and Identity* (1969). He considers not only how someone can develop a deviant identity (a frequent event), but how someone with a deviant identity can develop a normal identity, a less frequent event.

    Normal-smiths are those relatively rare persons or organized endeavors who assume that a person categorized as deviant is capable of rapid and wholesale change; that he or she is essentially capable of becoming "normal." The term normal-smith denotes the craftsmanship involved in imputing normality to a person labeled deviant and helping him or her assume normality.

    Lofland writes of both unusual individuals who are normal-smiths and organized endeavors of normal-smiths. Lay normal-smiths are exemplified by those employers who assume an ex-prisoner or recovered drug addict can go straight and gives the person a job. He gives two examples of organized normal-smiths: evangelical Christian groups, who in regarding all human beings as sinners, believe that therefore everyone can be saved, and self-help groups, such as Alcoholics Anonymous. AA regards the alcoholic as a person who is never able to drink alcohol normally and thus has a deviant characteristic, but the recovering alcoholic is capable of fast and dramatic change and can assume a normal identity in other respects.

2. To further complicate the issue of defining self-help, the "self" in self-help does not necessarily refer to an individual human being. It can refer to another social unit, such as a community, country, or state. In political parlance, "self-help" often refers to a legal entity like a county or city that is expected to finance or initiate its own projects. Discussions occur on the federal level about states and

communities engaging in self-help; what is meant is that the federal government will not finance or develop the project, and the lower-level political unit should finance and carry out the project with its own resources.

3. Self-help groups and support groups have limited appeal, and attract only a small proportion of the people who have access to them—even when people are informed about the groups' value and their benefits are explained (see Kaufmann, Schulberg, and Schooler 1994; Levy and Derby 1992; Medvene et al. 1994; and Weinberg et al. 1996). Benjamin Gottlieb and Larry Peters (1991) found that those who attend self-help groups are from the same population of people who join voluntary associations.

4. Self-help resource centers or clearinghouses are important mediating organizations between self-help/mutual aid, on the one hand, and the public, professionals, and governments, on the other hand. See Brock and Aronowitz (1982), Madara (1986, 1992, 1995), Madara, Kalafat, and Miller (1988), White and Madara (1998), and Wollert (1990). For information about Canadian clearinghouses, see D'Asaro (1994), Todres (1995), Todres and Hagarty (1993).

5. The diversity of self-help groups, networks, and alliances is extensive but unmapped. For illustrations of the variety, see the *Resources for People with Facial Difference*, a publication of Let's Face It, a network of individuals with only a few groups as nodes of the network (Let's Face It 1997). *Genetics Support Groups: Volunteers and Professionals as Partners* (Weiss et al. 1986) describes an alliance of various nonprofit health agencies, self-help and support groups, and conventional health foundations that deal with genetic disorders. In "Differences between National Self-Help Organizations and Local Self-Help Groups," in his edited book *Working with Self-Help*, Thomas Powell (1990) describes and compares nationally organized self-help efforts with local one-of-a-kind groups.

Self-help agencies are another variety of self-help group, although they are not referred to as such in the literature. Alfred Katz and Carl Maida (1990) discuss self-help agencies for people with disabilities, such as Independent Living Centers. Social model recovery programs for alcoholics and drug addicts are often self-help agencies (see Borkman 1983; Crawford 1997; Kaskutas and McLellan 1998; and Shaw and Borkman 1990).

Computer online chat rooms, support groups, and bulletin boards have proliferated during the last few years (Madara 1997, 1998; White and Madara 1998). For examples of studies of online groups, see Gerald Gold's "Chronic Illness and Disability in an Electronic Support Group" (1995), or Wende Phillips's "A Comparison of Online, E-Mail, and In-Person Self-Help Groups Using Adult Children of Alcoholics as a Model," <http://www.rider.edu/~suler/psycyber/acoa.html> (1996).

6. The 12-step recovery began to be represented in popular culture by the late 1980s: in the "John Laroquette" television show, John admits his problem with alcohol and goes to Alcoholics Anonymous; Cagney of "Cagney and Lacey" goes to AA as well. Cartoons mimic the 12-step introduction: "Hi, I'm Jeff, and I'm a Buffalo fan"; the audience responds, "Hi, Jeff!" and the caption reads "Buffalo Fans Anonymous"—the scene refers to the disheartened fans of the perennial Super Bowl–losing football team, the Buffalo Bills. The codependents' movement spawned jokes such as "if Decartes were codependent, he would have said 'you think, therefore I am.'" See Cavanaugh (1998), Rapping (1997), and Room and Greenfield (1993) for more discussion of the 12-step recovery movement.

Within weeks after the Persian Gulf War began in 1991, thousands of support groups were convened by family and friends of military personnel or by professionals. The social technology of operating a support group had clearly diffused throughout the American culture. Even skeptical physicians have found evidence that support groups may keep women with breast cancer living up to eighteen months longer than a matched control group that has equivalent medical care but no support group (Speigel et al. 1989).

7. This typology was inspired by the work of Mark Lefton and William R. Rosengren, who characterized hospitals and other formal agencies by the length of time the patient was expected to stay (longitudinal dimension) and the extent of the patient's biography (laterality); Lefton and Rosengren (1966); Rosengren and Lefton (1969). The two variables in the typology are the critical ones that affect the kinds of organizational issues the group faces, the extent to which a community or network is likely to evolve around the group, and how different views of the same problem lead to important differences in organizations.

8. For classic formulations of stigma and societal labeling, see Erving Goffman's *Stigma* (1963). See also Becker (1963), Lemert (1951), and Lofland (1969). Howard Becker borrowed Everett C. Hughes's concept of master and subordinate status and applied it to social deviants; a master status overrides all other statuses that a person has (1963, 32–36). For more recent work, see Conrad and Schneider (1980), Fox (1986), and Goode (1997).

9. Sociological and historical analysis of the professions, especially the medical profession, has flourished since the 1960s. See Abbott (1988), Cockerham (1998), Friedson (1970a, b, 1973), Starr (1982), Stevens (1971), and Turner (1995).

10. Self-help groups have been lumped with other emotionally expressive phenomena and criticized in general terms (Hughes 1993; Mestrovic 1997), or have sometimes been attacked without substantiating data (Kaminer 1993; Kasl 1992; Katz and Liu 1991; and Rapping 1997). Thoughtful criticism, including an examination of the limitations of self-help/mutual aid, is offered by such observers as Mark Chesler (1990), Linda Kurtz (1997), and Robert Wuthnow (1994).

11. I am following the model of some feminists (see Goldberger 1996; Goldberger et al. 1986; and Harding 1996) who deliberately choose the terminology "knowing" and "knowledge" instead of the language of "voices" because it deals with epistemological questions: To whom do I listen? What counts for me as evidence? How do I know what it true? What is authority? How do I know that I know? These questions also apply to self-help/mutual aid organizations. Given a society in which the scientific and helping professions are such privileged epistemic communities (that is, their knowledge and methods are socially valued as the basis of truth), how do patients and clients who undergo wrenching experiences and who cope with these issues as a collective come to value what they learn? How do they come to know that they have experiential knowledge about their situation? Empowerment has become such a popular term that its meaning has become diluted. Effective self-help/mutual aid, however, can and does empower (in the strongest sense of the term) self-helpers as collectivities to rise above the stigmatized or negative view of their disease or predicament and substitute a liberating meaning perspective. For more discussion of this issue, see Borkman (1976, 1983, 1984, 1990a) and Schubert and Borkman (1994).

Some social scientists use the terminology of "voices" to indicate the perspective of a minority of people and the verbalization of their perspective. This terminology can imply that the world is a relativistic one in which each person's opinion of what is true is as good as any other's. In these terms, the bystander who has no personal experience with coronary bypass surgery has a similarly weighted "voice" as the cardiologist who performs the operation or the patient who undergoes the surgery and recovers in Mended Hearts, a self-help group that is a collective of thousands of patients with similar experiences. The concept of "voice" finesses the issue of societal power and authority. The terminology of "knowledge" and "knowing," in contrast, conveys what I see as the reality of many self-help groups. They do not just *think* they know how to deal with their problem. In the sense of a satisfactory way to live, they come to *know* they know.

12. Studies of narratives or stories include Brody (1987), Bruner (1986, 1990), Polkinghorn (1988), Pollner and Stein (1996), Rappaport (1993), and Sarbin (1986).

13. Another meaning of "professional" that is not used here contrasts professionals and amateurs: the professional works for pay, while the amateur contributes services. For more discussion of definitions and characteristics of various professions, see Eliot Friedson's *The Professions and Their Prospects* (1973). Both the fact that professions are careers with varying levels of prestige and renumeration and the way in which concerns about careers influence practice are discussed by Abbott (1988), Cockerham (1998), Friedson (1970a, 1970b, 1973), and Starr (1982).

Chapter 2 *Experiential Learning*

1. The mind/body split is being questioned and rejected today by many philosophers, scientists, and social scientists (see Bateson 1979; Goldberger 1996; Goldberger et al. 1996; Reed 1996b; and Taylor 1995). Although the spiritual has been ignored in social science, indications are that it is being revived (see Chapter 7). Even the popular media claims that science is showing an interest in the spiritual: the cover story of the July 20, 1998, issue of *Newsweek* magazine was entitled "Science Finds God" (Begley 1998).

2. Schmitz distinguishes among privacy, familiarity, and intimacy (1986, 40). Privacy is an effort to block another person from knowing something about us. Familiarity connotes knowledge that gradually develops based on the accumulation of details about a person or thing that leads us to accept a certain pattern of behavior. Intimacy, however, connotes a relationship of some depth between people.

3. See James Campbell's discussion of the collegial relationship of George Herbert Mead, John Dewey, and William James and the stimulating exchange of ideas at the University of Chicago (1995). See also James (1978) and G. H. Mead ([1934] 1962) for more detail.

4. Psychoneuroimmunology is a developing field of interdisciplinary study that establishes relationships between the brain, behavior, and the immune system. See Ader and Cohen (1993); Ader, Felten, and Cohen (1991); Kennedy, Kiecolt-Glaser, and Glaser (1988); Kiecolt-Glaser and Glaser (1995); Kiecolt-Glaser et al. (1992, 1995); Maier, Watkins, and Fleshner (1994); and O'Leary (1990).

5. Rachel Naomi Remen is medical director and cofounder of the Commonwealth Cancer Help Program in Bolinas, California. Her article "On Defining Spirit" has been the most popular reprint in twenty years of publishing at the *Noetic Sciences Review*. The term "noetic" comes from the Greek word nous, which refers to mind, intelligence, or ways of knowing. The Institute of Noetic Sciences is a membership organization devoted to research and education on developing a science of mind and consciousness.

6. Existential concerns and questions about one's basic humanity are found in the Caring Group on Stuttering, described in chapters 1 and 5 and throughout this book. In addition, Chesler and Chesney (1995) and Chesler and Yoak (1984) discuss parents of children with cancer, and Riches and Dawson (1996) discuss bereaved parents.

7. The chemist Michael Polyani (1958, 1969), Gregory Bateson (1979), and Nancy

Dixon (1994) discuss how much of our knowledge is tacit or outside everyday consciousness.

8. The health belief model has been developed and tested over a period of twenty-five years. On its origins, see Rosenstock (1974); on its use in research, see Cummings, Becker, and Maile (1980), Janz and Becker (1984), and Taylor (1995).

9. The comparison of the didactic teaching of 12-step ideas in the hospital program and the experientially based teaching in the social model recovery program is discussed in Kaskutas, Marsh, and Kohn (1998). On the larger study comparing a hospital treatment program with the social model recovery program, see Kaskutas and McLellan (1998).

10. Julian Rappaport (1993) focuses on the community-level narrative which is similar to my term "meaning perspective." See also Humphreys and Rappaport (1994), and Kennedy and Humphreys (1994).

11. Jack Mezirow (1991) uses the term "meaning perspective" in a way similar to the way that I use it, although I did not consciously borrow it from him. He describes the terms other authors use for similar ideas in chapter 2 of *Transformative Dimensions of Adult Learning* (1991). Jerome Bruner has been interested in "folk psychology"—the common sense of cultures or the set of ideas and beliefs, more or less connected, about how human beings should and do operate, think, and behave in various situations. The anthropologists' examination of nonindustrial societies and their peoples are the best-studied "folk psychologies" (Bruner 1990, 33–36).

12. Paulo Freire's *Pedagogy of the Oppressed* (1970) is probably the best-known example of radical community-level education. Freire worked with illiterate peasants, helping them learn to read by using a methodology that increased their physical consciousness about how they were being oppressed.

13. As a highly technical area of psychology, self-efficacy and other aspects of social learning theory are tested in empirical research. Various conceptual distinctions are being made about facets of self-efficacy (see Bandura 1995), and scales for measuring these aspects have been developed and used. Perhaps hundreds of research studies have tested and refined these ideas. Researchers interested in applying self-efficacy theory to self-help groups would have a fruitful area of inquiry. See Taylor (1995) for findings that are useful in health psychology.

14. Feminist philosophers and social researchers have developed theories of knowledge that argue that what is regarded as valid knowledge is that which has been developed by the social groups in power, namely men or, more specifically, white men, and that the viewpoints and bodies of knowledge developed by women (part of the Other) have been ignored and rendered invisible (Harding 1991, 105). As an alternative, feminist philosophers and social scientists have been developing feminist epistemology, especially the feminist standpoint (see Anderson and Collins 1995; Goldberger et al. 1996; and Harding 1996). A standpoint is not simply an interested position that is interpreted as a bias, but an achieved set of assumptions, understandings, and body of knowledge that is liberated from the dominant viewpoint of those in power. A standpoint is in effect a transforming point of view that is free from the dominant, male-centered one. It differs from a perspective that is not an achievement and can be had by "opening one's eyes."

Sandra Harding (1991, 123) argues that standpoint theories must be grounded in an objective location, women's lives, as the place to begin rather than women's experiences. Experience itself is shaped by social location; women used to regard assaults by their husbands for sex as within the expected range of experience of heterosexual sex; women had to learn to define those sexual assaults within marriage as rape. What actual women experience is often within an unliberated viewpoint; women are at different stages of awareness, and some accept being subordinated or abused by men as "natural." Accordingly, women's words or experiences are not reliable grounds for knowledge or claims about nature and social relations.

I have adapted Harding's ideas of liberating standpoint to the self-help/mutual aid context. I prefer the term "liberating meaning perspective," because it is more active. Standpoint connotes a static and even dogmatic position. Harding's idea that experience "lies" is important, as in the example above—the traditional viewpoint is that women cannot be raped by their husbands because they are the property of their husbands, but from a liberating meaning perspective, however, it is unacceptable for men to sexually assault their wives.

15. See Robertson (1988) and *Twelve Steps and Twelve Traditions* (Alcoholics Anonymous [1952] 1974) for discussion of the positive life-enhancing aspects of 12-step programs.

16. The compatibility between an individual's worldview and the meaning perspective of the group is part of the person-group fit as described in Ken Maton's schema (1993). Although this is recognized as important, little research has been done. For more discussion, see Medvene et al. 1994, and the discussion in chapter 6.

17. The voluntary and nonprofit sector has become a distinct field of study and practice. Over forty colleges and universities have programs in nonprofit management. Independent Sector is an association that represents philanthropic and nonprofit organizations. The Association for Research on Nonprofit Organizations and Voluntary Action (ARNOVA), previously the Association for Voluntary Action Research (AVAR), is an interdisciplinary professional association of academics and practitioners that holds an annual conference and publishes the *Nonprofit and Voluntary Sector Quarterly* (previously the *Journal of Voluntary Action Research*). Other professional associations have developed internationally, and two other journals (*Voluntas* and *Nonprofit Management and Leadership*) are devoted to the area. Sociologists, economists, urban planners, historians, lawyers, social workers, organizational analysts, and many other people study the voluntary sector. See Gray (1991), Hodgkinson et al. (1989), Lohmann (1992), Mason (1996), Milofsky (1988), O'Neill (1989), W. Powell (1987), Salamon and Anheier (1994), Smith (1997a, b), Von Til (1988), and Weisbrod (1988).

Chapter 3   *The Societal Context*

1. See Katz and Bender (1976a, 1990) and Riessman and Carroll (1995) for discussions of how loosened support systems and inadequate formal services hastened the development of self-help groups.

2. Cofiguration occurs for many immigrants. Many who immigrated to the United States in the early 1900s faced lives very different from those of their forebears. In its simplest form, the cofigurative culture is one in which there are no grandparents present to teach the past or to reinforce the traditional ways of viewing things (M. Mead 1970, 34). Or, when they are present, grandparents have lost their authority. A cofigurative culture has been institutionalized among age mates when a "teenage" culture can be seen (M. Mead 1970, 45). Mead believes that the culturewide effects of cofiguration could be felt by 1900 in the United States, with the increased emphasis on the nuclear family and the diminished authority of grandparents. She added that by 1920, style-setting was beginning to be handed over to the mass media.

3. See Conrad and Schneider (1980), Fox (1986), and Zola (1972), for a discussion of medicalization and demedicalization.

4. The concept follows Paul Starr's (1982) idea of "cultural authority," which refers to institutionalized authority to define reality, to make judgments of meaning and value, to name things, and to have these constructions of meaning and value regarded as valid and true. His historical and sociological analysis of the rising power of the medical profession from the 1920s to the 1950s shows how physicians accrued cultural authority in conjunction with their medical authority.

5. See Chesler (1991) for an excellent analysis of how self-helper consumers have mobilized to improve professional practice and make other social changes. For other discussions of the impact of the civil rights movement, the anti–Vietnam War movement, the consumers' movement, and the women's movement on activism in self-help groups, see Borkman (1997), Chesler and Chesney (1995), Emerick (1991, 1996), Fox (1986), Kallick (1994), Katz (1993), McKnight (1994), Neighbors, Elliot, and Gant (1990), Nelson (1994), Nussbaum (1990), Riessman and Carroll (1995), Withorn (1994), and Zola (1987).

6. On the women's movement and its contributions to self-help and health, see Howes and Allina (1994), N. Gottlieb (1992), Hicks and Borkman (1988), Miller (1988), Rapping (1997), and Withorn (1994).

Chapter 4 **Professionals, Agencies, and the Commons**

1. Ambiguity and fuzziness in analyzing data and reporting findings about professional participation in self-help groups is illustrated by Morton Lieberman and Lonnie Snowden's 1993 article on assessing the prevalence and characteristics of members of self-help group participants. Using a sample of the more than three thousand self-help groups listed in the database of the California Self-Help Center at the University of California, Los Angeles, data indicated that 62 percent of the groups are led by paid professionals, 18 percent by voluntary professionals, and the remainder by members. The authors conclude that the image of member-run self-help groups does not fit the empirical reality they found in the data. However, no definition of the criteria used by the California Self-Help Center's for entering a group into the database was given. Perhaps the survey database included professionally led support groups as well as self-help groups, without distinguishing between them. Self-help resource centers often have explicit and clear criteria for what kinds of groups are allowed in their database of "self-help groups," and these are described in publications. Barbara White and Edward Madara (1998), for example, describe the criteria for inclusion in their database. The Self-Help Resource Center of Metropolitan Toronto defines its criteria in the *Mutual Aid Guide* (1994); it has a separate section for professionally led support groups.

2. Carl Milofsky (1987, 1988) suggests the key distinction between providing resources and exerting authority to control self-help groups. The resource-dependence model of organizational theory begins with the assumption that no organization can generate all of the resources it needs. It further assumes that organizations actively make decisions about resources and respond to environmental conditions. (See Aldrich and Pfeffer 1976; Hall 1996; Hasenfeld 1972; and Morgan 1997.) The model can be applied to self-help groups. Even groups that need minimal resources, such as 12-step/12-tradition groups, need potential members who are voluntarily willing to participate. The 12-step/12-tradition groups require few resources and are "self-supporting through their own contributions." They generate many of their own resources (except for members) from their membership. AA and other 12-tradition groups even limit the size of contributions members can make in a year, "decline outside contributions," and do not accept legacies (Alcoholics

Anonymous [1952] 1974). With these resources, they "rent" space to hold meetings in churches, government buildings, hospitals, and other social service or community agencies; they buy coffee (and other refreshments) and make it themselves. AA's national office is a publishing house that sells local groups copies of its literature. AA groups do depend upon professionals and treatment agencies to send potential members to them. At the other extreme are self-help agencies that require moderate to extensive resources, usually from governments or foundations, in order to maintain physical facilities and to pay staff to provide services to clients.

3. With these important publications self-help groups were clearly named as such. For more information, see Caplan and Killilea (1976), Gartner and Riessman (1977), Katz and Bender (1976), Lieberman and Borman (1976), and Robinson and Henry (1977).

4. Robert Emerick (1989, 1991, 1996) studied a national sample of 104 self-help groups for former mental patients and identified the variations in their ideologies. James Petersen and Gerald Markle (1979a, b) describe the laetrile groups.

5. Consumers of mental hospital services who participate in self-help groups have fewer repeat hospitalizations than those who do not participate (Edmunson, Bedell, et al. 1982; Humphreys 1997; Kennedy 1990; and L. Kurtz 1988). Studies of self-helpers who use professional services appropriately are described in Humphreys (1997), L. Kurtz (1997), Taylor (1995), and Taylor et al. (1986).

6. "Other" is a term used by feminists to refer to any stereotypical and categorical dualistic thinking that separates "We" from the "Other"; the other implies a devalued and perhaps stigmatized category. For further discussion, see Belenky, Bond, and Weinstock (1997).

7. Many researchers and other professionals "came out of the closet" in the 1980s and 1990s in the sense that they revealed their illnesses, flaws, and addictions. For example, the recently-deceased sociologist Irving Zola spoke about the polio and auto accident that left him limping and with chronic physical disabilities in his book *Missing Pieces: A Chronicle of Living with a Disability* (1982). He also helped to develop the Society for Disability Studies, many of whose members are researchers with disabilities. The anthropologist Robert F. Murphy wrote about his diminishing physical capacity and reduced sense of self owing to an encroaching brain tumor in *The Body Silent* (1990).

8. In psychology, see Davison and Neale (1998) for a categorization of major clinical orientations. For "new age" psychology outside the mainstream that explicitly incorporates the spiritual, see Carroll (1993).

9. The community psychology division (27) of the American Psychological Association hosts an interest group of more than one hundred participants who have an interest in developments within self-help. Division 27 sponsors the peer-reviewed *American Journal of Community Psychology*, which publishes a relatively large number of articles on self-help/mutual aid.

Community psychologists who view self-help/mutual aid within a broad context include Julian Rappaport (1993), who has pioneered in applying the study of narratives to self-help/mutual aid and, among other contributions, understands the "community vision." Keith Humphreys (1997) also understands the "community vision" and, among other contributions (Humphreys and Rappaport 1994), is studying how affiliation with 12-step mutual aid groups affects friendship networks in the community and how friendship networks affect abstinence among recovering substance abusers (Humphreys and Noke 1997). Francine Lavoie and others (1994) have considered ethical concerns about (more powerful) professionals relating to (weaker) self-help groups. Kenneth Maton (1993) proposes multilevel models of research on self-help/mutual aid that locate groups within their community context and does comparative studies of groups. Louis Medvene (1984) understands that the helping relationships are gifts, not contractual exchanges, and studies dual-status professionals. Gregory Meissen directs a self-help resource center and is exploring how self-help/mutual aid can relate to managed care (Meissen and Warren 1997).

10. The impact of requirements for accountability from funding sources can shape nonprofit program services. See Gronbjerg (1992) for more information about human service agencies. Bradford Gray (1991) analyzes changes in nonprofit hospitals resulting from the increasing competition of corporate-style hospitals; Lisa Dicke and Steven Ott (1997) and Steven Smith and Michael Lipsky (1993) speak in more general terms about the issues.

11. References to self-help agencies (which are not named as such) for recovery from substance abuse or physical disabilities include Kaskutas and McLellan (1998), Katz and Maida (1990), Shaw and Borkman (1990), and Zola (1987). Consumer-run mental health services are summarized in Davidson and others (1997). See chapter 1, note 5, above.

12. See Borkman (1997) for an examination of the way in which public health policy includes or excludes self-help/mutual aid and what impact this has on resources received by self-help resource centers from governments and foundations in Canada and the United States. See Jemmott (1997) for one of the few discussions of foundations' relationships with self-help/mutual aid. See Hedrick, Isenberg, and Martini (1992) for a description of attempts to influence federal agencies, the media, and health and human service agencies to value and use self-help/mutual aid following the Surgeon General's Workshop on Self-Help and Public Health .

13. Self-help resource centers often take the phase-out approach. Professionals are viewed as important to help initiate groups in some situations, but training sessions for professionals include planning how to help members "own" the group from the beginning, and how the professional can gradually phase out active control. Judy Wilson (1995), at the Nottingham self-help center in England, takes this approach, as do Edward Madara (1998) in New Jersey and the Self-Help Resource Centre of Metro Toronto.

14. Parents Anonymous (Willen 1984), with its dual authority structure (experiential and professional), has tended to become more professionalized according to Linda Kurtz (1997). Wounded clients who are new to receiving help may prefer professional help and regard it to be safer as well as more knowledgeable than self-help/mutual aid (see Medvene et al. 1994).

15. Relatively extensive and important research on the individual benefits of participation in self-help groups as well as the dynamics of group functioning has been conducted since Morton Lieberman and Leonard Borman (1976) declared that no adequate study of group effectiveness had been done. Using psychotherapy from the 1970s as a gold standard against which the benefits of self-help/mutual aid were measured, research has shown that self-help/mutual aid has significant benefits for involved members, the benefits are not well captured by using the measuring instruments designed for psychotherapy, and self-help/mutual aid has other benefits and impacts than does psychotherapy.

Significant increases in knowledge have resulted. As illustrations of this, see Borkman (1991), Chesler and Chesney (1995), Emerick (1991, 1996), Humphreys (1997), Katz (1993), Katz et al. (1992), L. Kurtz (1997), Lavoie, Borkman, and Gidron (1994), Levy (1976), Levy and Derby (1992), Lieberman and Borman (1979), T. Powell (1990, 1994), and Riessman and Carroll (1995).

16. Seymour Sarason, in an insightful book, *The Creation of Settings and the Future of Societies* (1972), makes similar arguments about being a prisoner of one's worldview. Professionals have a certain way of thinking of which they are often unaware; these thought patterns lead to the repetition of past behaviors. For example, Sarason speaks of the way in which the solutions to problems arrived at by professionals usually end up being those that involve professionals like themselves; for substantial change to occur, their mind set would have to change. Sarason says that the "meaning perspective" of professionals propels them to problem-solve within a narrow range of ideas that includes their own definition of problems and their own type of services as the preferred solution. Our frame of reference locks us into a restricted way of identifying and responding to problems, a way grounded in our training and experiences. Professionals are still formulating self-help/mutual aid from within the prism or paradigm of professional services. A few maverick professionals see beyond their worldview (Farquharson 1995).

17. Descriptions and analyses of tensions between self-help and professional systems can be found in Borkman (1990b), Chesler (1990), Chesler and Chesney (1995), Audrey Gartner (1997), Lenrow and Burch (1981), Stewart (1990a), Stewart et al. (1994), and Todres (1982).

Chapter 5 *Evolution of People Who Stutter*

1. I conducted four studies of self-help groups for people who stutter. The first was a study of the Caring Group through one and one-half years of participant observation and a survey of previous attendees; the study was supported by a 1970–1971 Catholic University Faculty Research Grant (Borkman 1973, 1976). The second study, a mail questionnaire about the organizational aspects of eighteen groups for people who stutter in the United States, New Zealand, Sweden, and Holland, was supported by a 1972–1973 grant from the National Institutes of Mental Health (Borkman 1974, 1975b; Borkman and Hickey 1978). Third, a comparative study of three self-help groups—AA, an ostomy association, and the Caring Group on Stuttering—was supported by a 1977 faculty research grant from George Mason University. Seasoned members from each organization were interviewed about their experiential knowledge and the group's meaning perspective (Borkman 1979, 1984). Fourth, a mail questionnaire survey of the organizational aspects of thirty-three self-help groups for people who stutter in the United States was done in 1983 (Shaw, Shaw, and Borkman 1985; Borkman, Shaw, Shaw, and Hickey 1985). I maintained intermittent contacts with leaders of various national and local groups and conducted some follow-up interviews with them in 1993 and in 1998.

2. Many studies of self-help groups have interviewed participants and report selected segments of their stories in published works. For examples, see Chesler and Chesney (1995), Kennedy and Humphreys (1994), and Silverman and Smith (1984).

3. Marty Jezer (1997) writes about his experiences with the Hollins College fluency precision shaping program, the Edinburgh Masker, various speech therapies, psychotherapy, and self-help groups for people who stutter.

4. For discussion of the nonavoidance approach to stuttering see Sheehan (1965, 1970) and Van Riper (1963, 1971).

Chapter 6 *A Liberating Meaning Perspective*

1. The criteria a researcher or observer uses to determine the stage of a group's meaning perspective is relevant in empirical research. For the Caring Group on Stut-

tering, an inadequate amount of information over the seventeen-year period was available to determine exactly when the fledgling stage stopped and the second stage began. The four studies were done in 1970–71, 1972–73, 1977, and 1983; see note 1 in chapter 5 for a description of the studies and the data that were available. The timetables of the stages given here are rough approximations based on the available data.

The Caring Group's liberating meaning perspective was not codified in a central place. Bits and pieces of it were found in newsletters, letters of officers to members, the bylaws, articles of incorporation, and the like. The meaning perspective was mostly carried by the stories and lives of its members, especially committed long-term members who exemplified it in the way they had changed their lives. In that sense, a meaning perspective is a "living story," so to speak; as the members change in a group, the "living story" will change to reflect the viewpoints of the current members. Some people are trailblazers whose visions and ideas are introduced but have not been accepted by regular seasoned members of the group. Ellen and Dick in the Caring Group were two trailblazers who often led the group in terms of new ideas.

Measuring experiential authority or seeing its manifestation in a group is also critical in research. Experiential authority concerning the issue of not having friends or social events might have been exhibited as follows: if a speech therapist criticized them for holding social events in 1976 when they had a mature meaning perspective, they would have confidently disagreed based on their evidence from experience about how useful social events and friendships were to the personal recovery of individuals and to the maintenance of the organization.

An analysis of the conversation of seasoned members of the group is a good way to identify in what stage the meaning perspective is in. They state that they know certain things and are willing to defend their ideas to professionals or other authority figures. The leaders, old-timers, and veteran members of the group are more likely to be the carriers of the group's perspective and idioculture than are newcomers, peripheral participants, or occasional drop-ins. The perspective of the group is, in general, known and transmitted by the seasoned members through their stories, their behavior and way of life, and the group's writings in newsletters, and so forth. But an observer cannot assume that the stories of a specific individual reflect the group's meaning perspective in toto. A story also reflects the personal opinions and experiences of the person expressing it, and may not coincide exactly with that of the group.

2. The multitude of theories about stuttering and its therapies that the Caring Group dealt with are described by Bloodstein (1958), Sheehan (1965, 1970), Jezer (1997), and Van Riper (1963, 1971).

3. An interiorized stutterer or inner stutterer may be fluent but be afraid he will stutter; some are called "phobic normal speakers" (see Sheehan 1970, 345).

4. David Mason (1996, xi) defines expressive behavior as "action for direct rather than indirect gratification. It is play for the sake of the play; work for the sake of the work; energy spent for the sake of the spending." He shows that nonprofit and voluntary organizations are different from commercial enterprises because of their value orientation—their expressive goals and related social technologies. He maintains that management techniques that promote efficiency in a business are inappropriate in expressively oriented voluntary associations composed of volunteers. Roger Lohmann (1992) makes similar points in *The Commons*, of which self-help/mutual aid is a part.

5. Informal organization refers to the personal relationships and contacts of friendship

or exchange that individuals develop in an organization; the informal organization "oils the machinery" of the formal organization and can cross hierarchical levels or functional units. See Mason (1996), Morgan (1986), Perrow (1986). Rosabeth Moss Kanter (1972) shows how commitment to relationships in a group affects the cohesiveness of the group and individuals' willingness to help maintain it.

6. Michael Hannah and John H. Freeman (1989) are known for having developed the population ecology version of organizations as open systems influenced by their environments.

Technology was defined in chapter 1 (see note 1) in a generic sense as the means or techniques to accomplish goals. In the organizational literature, the hypothesis is that the nature of the "raw material" on which the organization works determines the appropriate technology to be used, and the kind of technology shapes an appropriate organizational structure. For example, if the "raw material" processed by an organization is perceived to be uniform and predictable, then a mechanistic technology will be used that is compatible with a bureaucratic structure. "Raw material" that is perceived to be unpredictable and distinctive requires a more participatory organization as the workers need discretion to fashion the "raw material" into finished products.

While the technology argument was initiated for organizations dealing with material production, Charles Perrow (1986) adapted it to people-processing organizations. If the human beings as the "raw material" are perceived to be unpredictable or unique, then the tasks to work with them are nonroutine. Workers who do the work (for example, teach, nurse, or babysit) need discretion in order to deal with unpredictable clients. Perrow uses examples of custodial mental hospitals or ghetto schools that regard their charges as uniform and well understood, with the central task being the maintenance of order. A bureaucracy is an organizational form that can efficiently handle order in both the ghetto school and the custodial hospital. In contrast, a private school in a wealthy suburb may regard its students as unique and unpredictable with the goal being to mold the whole personality; an organizational structure that allows teachers leeway to give individual attention is needed—a more decentralized and participatory structure than a standard bureaucracy.

In self-help/mutual aid groups such as the Caring Group, the "raw material" is the member or participant who is being changed. In effect, self-help groups, in regarding their members as holistic human persons, implicitly regard themselves—the "raw material"—as distinctive and unpredictable. Furthermore, they assume that the "raw material" cannot be changed without its willing commitment and effort—the self-helper has to be actively involved. Thus, a participatory form of organization is a compatible, if not a necessary, structure.

Carl Milofsky (1987) points out that the "death" of a voluntary association, community organization, or self-help group cannot automatically be equated with failure as is the tendency in thinking about businesses. Mark Hager (1997) more recently raised the same issue and argues that member-benefit associations, including self-help groups, may disband when they accomplish their mission. I found this to be the case in my study of eighteen groups for people who stutter in 1972–73, although I did not know how to interpret the finding at the time (Borkman 1974). Members of a self-help group in New Zealand explained that they had disbanded their group because it had met their needs, and the members were going on to other personal goals rather than serve other people who stutter.

7. See chap. 2, note 16. Studies looking at the person-group fit of worldview include

Antze (1976), Luke, Roberts, and Rappaport (1993), and Medvene et al. (1994). Lee Kaskutas (1992, 1994) has an interesting sample of attendees to Women for Sobriety—many of whom had been to or continued to go to AA; she compares the beliefs of (1) those who first got sober in AA with (2) those who first got sober in Women for Sobriety, and then went to AA with (3) those who never went to AA.

8. Benjamin Gidron and Mark Chesler (1994) suggest that there are universal aspects of self-help/mutual aid as well as aspects distinctive to a society because of its culture, values and beliefs, government, and type of health and human services system. The cultural and societal similarities and differences in self-help/mutual aid are an important but very new area of research (see Borkman 1997; Chesler, Chesney and Gidron 1990; Lavoie, Borkman, and Gidron 1994; Oka 1994; Trojan et al. 1990; von Appen 1994; and Wong and Chan 1994).

Chapter 7   *Transforming Individual Perspectives*

1. Experiential learning occurs in many more contexts than just self-help groups. In professionally facilitated support groups as well as self-help groups, "victims" can work through their painful and wounding experiences and reflect upon them in a safe group context that provides various perspectives. Individuals can also go through the experiential learning process alone, with a self-help book or audiotape, with a regular support network of family and friends, or with professional therapy. Some individuals use writing, art, and other creative means as a vehicle for working through their experiences; we know little about creative processes and their effectiveness in experiential learning. But what kinds of understanding and insights do people reach who work through their experiences in various ways? People who learn with experiential peers are problem solving in a context that uses the power of the group to facilitate individual change with the advantage of multiple perspectives from the various participants. Studies of social psychology have found groups to be a most powerful facilitator of change in individuals (Johnson and Johnson 1997; Forsyth 1990).

2. Other adult education leaders have the same tendency to equate education with a formal institution that requires certified teachers (see Merriam and Caffarella 1991 or Thorpe, Edwards, and Hansons 1993). Others such as Long (1990) and Tuijnman and van der Kamp (1992) frame adult education within the wider community context.

3. The group climate concept has been extensively developed, tested, and applied to a wide variety of groups over many years. See the original conceptual development in Moos (1974). Linda Kurtz (1997) summarizes the findings of several studies of group climate in self-help groups; see also Perkins, Lafuze and Van Dusen (1994), who measured group climate in groups for the mentally ill. Rudolph Moos, John Finney, and Peg Maude-Griffon (1993) review the use and potential of group climate scales in self-help groups and psychotherapy groups.

4. See Gerald Gold's work (1995) on on-line computer groups for people with multiple sclerosis. Edward Madara's work (1997; see also White and Madara 1998) on computer on-line groups is extensive. The literature is expanding rapidly.

5. The types of stories people learn in self-help groups are described and categorized by Kennedy and Humphreys (1994), Pollner and Stein (1996), and Rudy (1986).

6. The idea that emotional resocialization and other behaviors are slow to change is described by Sandra Coyle (1996), implied by the findings of Kaskutas, Marsh, and Kohn (1998), and stated by self-helpers I have interviewed. Members of self-

help groups often say that they see changes in other members' attitudes and behavior over time. They need to know the person well, however, because many
changes are small, incremental, and difficult to detect. Members also report that
others recognize and comment on changes before they can see them in themselves;
individuals rely on others who know them to help record their progress (phase 4
of the cycle of learning).

7. Linda Kurtz (1997) summarizes the two types of models of affiliation and readiness for change. Each is a five-stage model. The affiliation model pertains to phases
of attachment to the self-help/mutual aid group, which in my terminology would
be equated with commitment to the group's meaning perspective. The readiness
to change is also a five-phase model: the first three phases involve contemplating
and preparing to change (see DiClemente 1993; Snow, Prochaska, and Rossi 1994).
Other models of stages of recovery from alcoholism and substance abuse have been
developed; see Brown (1993), Fowler (1993), and Straussner and Spiegel (1996).

8. Miriam Rodin (1985) looked at the amount and kinds of information that seasoned AA members gave to newcomers and found that it was appropriate for the
physical, mental, and emotional capacities of newly sober alcoholics. L. A.
Alibrandi (1982) also looked at the messages sponsors and old-timer AA members gave to novices and found that they were simple, uncomplicated, and within
the grasp of the detoxifying alcoholics who were undergoing extensive physiological
and psychological changes.

9. The feeling of not being alone but being understood is probably the most frequently
reported benefit of participating in self-help/mutual aid. The feeling that you do
not have to explain yourself is nicely described in Medvene and Krauss's 1985 ethnographic data on families of the mentally ill. For more discussion, see Riches and
Dawson (1996).

10. "Survivor" does not always imply working through some difficulty to achieve healing or recovery. Former mental patients often use the term "survivor" to indicate
that they have undergone a terrible ordeal in a mental hospital and barely survived; an analogy might be survivors of a collapsed mine tunnel. In my terminology those who use the term survivor to connote having undergone an ordeal
without any healing are in the "victim" phase.

11. Phillip Brickman and his colleagues (1982) distinguish between attribution of responsibility for a problem and attribution of responsibility for a solution to derive
four general models that specify what form people's behavior will take when they
try to help others (or themselves) and what form they expect the recipient's behavior to take. Brickman and his colleagues categorized AA and other 12-step programs as following the enlightenment model; in their view, the 12-step programs
believe their members are responsible for causing their problem but the responsibility for the solution lies with the group (1982, 374, 379). But then they contra-
dict themselves by implying that AA fits the compensatory model—in which the
member is not seen as responsible for having caused his/her alcoholism but is responsible for the solution; for example, alcoholics not only try to solve their own
problems, which they can do by accepting the discipline of the organization, but
increasingly take responsibility for helping other members with their drinking problems (1982, 377). The authors are saying that the low-solution category covers all
situations where more than the self, that is, the help of an organization, is needed.
They do not distinguish between voluntary participation, as in AA, and subjugat-
ing oneself to a cult. This apparent confusion about which of the four categories
fits AA occurs in part because the ideas of AA are more complex than can be
covered by their four models. AA distinguishes responsibility for causing the prob-

lem in an etiological sense from being responsible for the consequences of the problem. Thus alcoholics are regarded as not responsible for their alcoholism (that is, alcoholism is regarded as a biological disease that also has moral/spiritual, psychological, and social/environmental dimensions). Recovering alcoholics, however, are responsible for the "wreckage" they created during their active alcoholism, that is, the consequences of their alcoholic drinking. AA's steps 8 and 9 refer to making a list of people the alcoholic has harmed and becoming willing to make amends to them; amends as defined in the official literature goes beyond saying "I'm sorry" and includes making restitution whenever possible (Alcoholics Anonymous [1939] 1976, [1952] 1974).

In terms of responsibility for the solution, AA implicitly has a triangular partnership or interdependence model involving the self, the AA group, and a Higher Power. The recovering alcoholic is expected to do his or her part: stop drinking, "do the foot work," go to meetings, "easy does it but do it," work the 12 steps, have and consult with a sponsor or guide. Thus there are extensive efforts required of the individual in order to attain and maintain sobriety. However, the individual's willpower and effort alone is regarded as insufficient for sobriety according to AA literature; the person also needs a Higher Power (which is widely defined as the AA group, God, or some other power). Finally, a recovering alcoholic affiliates with the AA group for fellowship and support and to learn how to maintain sobriety.

The view presented here is consistent with the work of William Miller and Ernest Kurtz (1994), who point to the fact that many people confuse elements of other models (disease, moral, and personality models) with the basic tenets of the AA model as reflected in its writings. Miller and Kurtz divide the causes of alcoholism into moral/spiritual, biological, psychological, and social/environmental factors and explore the primary causal emphasis in each model. AA would say yes to all four potential causes, with primary emphasis on the spiritual. Miller and Kurtz also regard AA as categorizing alcoholism as a disease/illness, and as holding the alcoholic responsible for the past. They do not distinguish past consequences from etiology as I am doing. They also agree that the alcoholic has responsibilities in recovery, such as don't drink and work the steps, but the source of healing in recovery is God.

Chapter 8   *Self-Organizing Groups*

1. Max Weber compared traditionally and charismatically legitimated organizations with modern bureaucracies of his time and regarded the latter as more efficient. Weber's formulation of bureaucracy has predominated in the organizational literature.
2. The idea that bureaucracies can be instruments of power in which a ruling elite establishes an oligarchy was developed by Robert Michels, who wrote *Political Parties* in 1911 based on his study of the German Social Democratic Party and the socialist parties in France, Italy, and elsewhere. The "Iron Law of Oligarchy" is the idea that a small cadre of leaders become tyrannical, unresponsive to the membership, and deflect organizational goals in order to maintain their power. Iannello (1992) discusses alternatives to bureaucracies and argues that some feminists, among others who value participatory decision making, can operate within nonprofit organizations, modify the hierarchy, and maintain democratic governance. See Crawford (1997) for a description of a self-help agency for recovering substance abusers that developed an alternative management structure grounded in the

principles of the 12 traditions. The agency utilized experiential authority within the rational-legal hierarchical framework of a nonprofit organization.

3. The minimalist organization (see Aldrich et al. 1990) refers to an organization that is organized so that it has few resource requirements; many self-help/mutual aid organizations are minimalist organizations. Charles Bufe (1991) describes AA as an anarchist organization; see also Irving Gellman (1964).

4. Learning organization theory often focuses on individuals learning in the organization and applying cognitive models of learning (Simon 1991; Weick 1991; and Wheatley 1992). Gareth Morgan (1997) summarizes learning organization theory. Of interest here is collective learning, which Scott Cook and Dvora Yanow (1993) and Nancy Dixon (1994) include in their formulations.

5. While on a Fullbright Research Fellowship to the Voluntary Action Centre at York University in Toronto, I began a collaboration with Asaf Zohar. An expert in learning organization theory, he was looking for a case study of a nonprofit organization that exemplified self-organizing principles; he had been disappointed that the two nonprofit advocacy organizations he studied for his doctoral research had not been learning organizations. I was interested in understanding AA's structure from an organizational perspective, but none of the conceptual frameworks I knew fit AA. Asaf's theoretical acumen dovetailed with my knowledge of AA as a case study. See Zohar and Borkman (1997) and Borkman and Zohar (1997).

6. For studies of AA diversity, see Makela et al. (1996) for the study of AA in eight societies. Also see Kaskutas (1998), Makela (1993), Rosovsky et al. (1992), and Sutro (1989). Other studies of AA illustrate its diversity: Nan Robertson (1988) discusses AA in New York City, David Rudy (1986) studied AA members and their meetings in a mideastern city, and Milton Maxwell (1984) studied groups in Chicago and interviewed AA members from seven other states. Thomasina Borkman and John Messer (1996) interviewed AA members in San Francisco, Los Angeles, rural Pennsylvania, and the Washington, D.C., area.

7. The many types of AA meetings are described in DuPont and McGovern (1994), Robertson (1988), Maxwell (1984), and Makela et al. (1996). Basically, there are open meetings that anyone can attend, closed meetings for self-defined members or people who have a desire to stop drinking alcohol, and in urban areas meetings for special subgroups—women, gays and lesbians, atheists, and so forth.

8. D. W. Winicott's 1958 concept of a "holding environment," where it is safe for a person to struggle with issues of narcissism or immaturity and be transformed with the interactive help of another, is applied to AA meetings by Turnbull (1997) and by Straussner and Spiegel (1996); they apply psychological theories to personal changes of sober committed AA members.

9. The distinctive form of "dialogue" in AA and other 12-step/12-tradition meetings is described in Makela et al. (1996, chap. 11, "The AA Meeting as a Speech Event"). It is increasingly recognized that the AA language and culture are distinctive and not transparent to newcomers; novices need to be educated about the format and rules of meetings (for example, no cross-talk) and learn the culture (Pollner and Stein 1996). Two physicians, Robert DuPont and John McGovern (1994), wrote a book entitled *A Bridge to Recovery: An Introduction to 12-Step Programs* for professionals in which AA and other 12-step/12-tradition groups are explained and the preparation that clients need before attending AA is discussed.

10. See chap. 7, note 8.

11. For a discussion of AA groups with deviant ideas, or cults, see Messer (1994), Maxwell (1984), and Makela et al. (1996). See also *AA Comes of Age* (Alcoholics Anonymous 1957). Because AA is a voluntary association that is informally orga-

nized at the local level without membership lists or other documentation, and participation is self-selected, issues of sampling from an unknown population, lack of ready access to members, and other methodological problems limit the kinds of research that can be done (see McGrady and Miller 1993).

12. A number of theorists from various disciplines (Capra 1996; Gleick 1987; Goldstein 1994; Wheatley 1992) use analogies from biology and chemistry in developing ideas about organizations as self-organizing systems in which the focus is on processes of change, unfolding, and adaptation to turbulent environments rather than on static features such as structures. See Morgan (1986, 1997) for a synthesis of the major ideas.

13. The design principles of self-organizing systems are synthesized in Morgan (1986, 1997). The concept of redundancy of functions was developed by F. E. Emery and E. L. Trist (1965); see W. R. Ashby (1960) for a discussion of requisite variety. Ralph Stacey (1992) has contributed to the notion of minimum critical specifications.

Chapter 9 *Conclusion*

1. I think the critics of self-help groups are likely to see fledgling groups that are in the stage of complaining without constructive ways of dealing with the common problem, and then generalize from them to all of self-help/mutual aid.

References

Abbott, A. D. 1988. *The System of Professions: An Essay on the Division of Expert Labor*. Chicago: University of Chicago Press.

Ader, Robert, and Nicholas Cohen. 1993. Psychoneuroimmunology: Conditioning and stress. *Annual Review of Psychology* 44: 53–85.

Ader, Robert, D. L. Felton, and N. Cohen. 1991. *Psychoneuroimmunology*. 2nd ed. New York: Academic Press.

Alcoholics Anonymous. [1939] 1976. *Alcoholics Anonymous*. 3rd ed. New York: Alcoholics Anonymous Publishing.

———. [1952] 1974. *Twelve Steps and Twelve Traditions*. New York: Alcoholics Anonymous World Services.

———. 1955. *Alcoholics Anonymous*. 2nd ed. New York: Alcoholics Anonymous Publishing.

———. 1957. *Alcoholics Anonymous Comes of Age: A Brief History of A.A.* New York: Alcoholics Anonymous World Services.

———. 1970. Member's eye view of AA. New York: Alcoholics Anonymous Publishing.

———. 1994. *The A.A. Service Manual*. New York: Alcoholics Anonymous World Services.

Aldrich, Howard E., and Jeffrey Pfeffer. 1976. Environments of organizations. *Annual Review of Sociology* 2: 79–105.

Aldrich, Howard E., Udo Staber, Catherine Zimmer, and John Beggs. 1990. Minimalism and organizational mortality: Patterns of disbanding among U.S. trade associations, 1900–1983. In *Organizational Evolution: New Directions*, edited by Jitendra V. Singh. Newbury Park, Calif.: Sage Publications.

Alibrandi, L. 1982. The fellowship of Alcoholics Anonymous. In *Encyclopedic Handbook of Alcoholism*, edited by E. M. Pattison and E. Kaufman. New York: Gardner Press.

Anderson, Margaret L., and Patricia Hill Collins. 1995. Shifting the center and reconstructing knowledge. In *Race, Class, and Gender: An Anthology*, edited by Margaret Anderson and Patricia Hill Collins. Belmont, Calif.: Wadsworth Publishing.

Antze, Paul. 1976. The role of ideologies in peer psychotherapy groups. *Journal of Applied Behavioral Science* 12: 323–346.

Ashby, W. R. 1960. *An Introduction to Cybernetics*. London: Chapman and Hall.

Bandura, Albert. 1977. Self-efficacy: Toward a unifying theory of behavioral change. *Psychological Review* 84: 191–215.

———. 1986. *A Social Foundation of Thought and Action: A Social Cognitive Theory*. Englewood Cliffs, N.J.: Prentice-Hall.

———. 1993. Perceived self-efficacy in cognitive development and functioning. *Educational Psychologist* 28 (2): 117–148.

———, ed. 1995. *Self-Efficacy in Changing Societies*. New York: Cambridge University Press.

Barath, Arpad. 1990. Hypertension clubs in Croatia, Yugoslavia. In Katz, Alfred H., and Bender, Eugene I., eds., *Helping One Another: Self-Help Groups in a Changing World*. Oakland, Calif.: Third Party.

Barrows, David C. 1980. Informal interactions at an alcohol recovery home. Social Research Group, School of Public Health, University of California, Berkeley, California.

Bateson, Gregory. 1972. *Steps to an Ecology of Mind*. New York: Ballantine.

———. 1979. *Mind and Nature: A Necessary Unity*. New York: Ballantine.

Beattie, Melody. 1989. *Beyond Codependency: And Getting Better All the Time*. Center City, Minn.: Hazelden Foundation.

———. 1990. *Codependents' Guide to the Twelve Steps*. A Fireside/Parkside Recovery Book. New York: Simon and Schuster.

Becker, Howard. 1963. *Outsiders: Studies in the Sociology of Deviance*. New York: Free Press.

Begley, Sharon. 1998. Science finds God. *Newsweek*. July 20.

Belenky, Mary Field, Lynne A. Bond, and Jacqueline S. Weinstock. 1997. *A Tradition That Has No Name: Nurturing the Development of People, Families, and Communities*. New York: Basic Books.

Belenky, Mary Field, Blythe McVicker Clinchy, Nancy Rule Goldberger, and Jill Mattuck Tarule, eds. 1986. *Women's Ways of Knowing: The Development of Self, Voice, and Mind*. New York: Basic Books.

Bellah, Robert N., Richard Madsen, William Sullivan, Ann Swidler, and Steven M. Tipton. 1991. *The Good Society*. New York: Vintage Books.

Berger, Peter L., and Thomas T. Luckmann. 1967. *The Social Construction of Reality: A Treatise in the Sociology of Knowledge*. Garden City, N.Y.: Anchor Books.

Best, Joel, ed. 1989. *Images of Issues: Typifying Contemporary Social Problems*. New York: Aldine de Gruyter.

Bloodstein, Oliver. 1958. Stuttering as an anticipatory struggle reaction. In *Stuttering: A Symposium*, edited by Jon Eisenson. New York: Harper and Row.

Bloomfield, Kim. 1994. Beyond sobriety: The cultural significance of Alcoholics Anonymous as a social movement. *Nonprofit and Voluntary Sector Quarterly* 23 (1): 21–40.

Borkman, Thomasina J. 1973. Ingredients for survival: A profile of stutterers' self-help organizations. Final report to granting agency, National Institute for Mental Health.

———. 1974. A cross-cultural comparison of stutterers' self-help organizations. *New Zealand Speech Therapists' Journal* 29 (May): 6–16.

———. 1975a. Changing sex roles: Consciousness-raising groups as a vehicle of adult resocialization. *In Sociological Research Symposium V*, edited by J. Williams, A. Schwartzbaum, and R. Caney. Richmond, Va.: Virginia Commonwealth University.

————. 1975b. "Stutterers" self-help organizations: Emergence of group life among the stigmatized. *Sociological Research Symposium* V, edited by J. Williams, A. Schwartzbaum, and R. Caney. Richmond, Va.: Virginia Commonwealth University.

————. 1976. Experiential knowledge: A new concept for the analysis of self-help groups. *Social Science Review* 50: 445–455.

————. 1979. *Mutual Self-Help Groups: A Theory of Experiential Inquiry.* Rockville, Md.: National Institute on Alcohol Abuse and Alcoholism.

————. 1983. A social-experiential model in programs for alcoholism recovery: A research report on a new treatment design. Rockville, Md.: National Institute for Alcohol Abuse and Alcoholism, United States Department of Health and Human Services, publication no. (ADM) 83–1259.

————. 1984. Mutual self-help groups: Strengthening the selectively unsupportive personal and community networks of their members. In *The Self-Help Revolution*, edited by F. Reissman and A. Gartner. New York: Human Sciences Press.

————. 1990a. Experiential, professional, and lay frames of reference. In *Working with Self Help*, edited by Thomas J. Powell. Silver Spring, Md.: National Social Workers Press.

————. 1990b. Self-help groups at the turning point: Emerging egalitarian alliances with the formal health care system. *American Journal of Community Psychology* 18 (2): 321–331.

————. 1991. Introduction to the Special Issue. *American Journal of Community Psychology* 19 (5): 643–650.

————. 1993. Conceptualizing mutual aid self-help as commons, not alternatives to professional services. Paper presented at the 22nd annual conference of the Association for Research on Nonprofit Organizations and Voluntary Action, October 28, Toronto.

————. 1997. How public policy affects the development of self-help and mutual aid resources: a comparison of U.S. and Canada. Revision of paper presented at the conference of the International Society for Third Sector Research, July 19, 1996, Mexico City.

Borkman, Thomasina, and Anthony Hickey. 1978. Comparative study of stutterers' self-help organizations and their community relations. Paper presented at the meeting of the Association for Voluntary Action Research, October 7, Toronto.

Borkman, Thomasina, and John G. Messer. 1996. The role of mutual aid self-help in building social capital. Paper presented at the Silver Anniversary Conference of ARNOVA, November 7–9, New York.

Borkman, Thomasina, and Maria Parisi. 1995. The role of self-help groups in fostering a caring society. In *Care and Community in Modern Society*, edited by Paul G. Schervisch, Virginia A. Hodgkinson, Margaret Gates, and associates. San Francisco: Jossey-Bass.

Borkman, Thomasina, Mark Shaw, Richard Shaw, and Anthony Hickey. 1984. Survivability of self-help groups for persons who stutter: A discriminant analysis. Paper presented at the meeting of the Association of Voluntary Action Scholars, October, Blacksburg, Va.

Borkman, Thomasina, and Asaf Zohar. 1996. The culture of experiential learning in Alcoholics Anonymous.

Borman, Leonard. 1979. Characteristics of development and growth. In *Self-Help Groups for Coping with Crisis*, edited by Morton A. Lieberman and Leonard Borman. San Francisco: Jossey-Bass.

————. 1982. Leadership in self-help/mutual aid groups. In *Citizen Participation* 3 (3): 30–31.

Bradshaw, John. 1990. *Homecoming: Reclaiming and Championing Your Inner Child*. New York: Bantam Books.

———. 1996. *The Family: A New Way of Creating Solid Self-Esteem*. Deerfield Beach, Fla.: Health Communications, Inc.

Brickman, Philip, Vita Carulli Rabinowitz, Jurgis Karuza, Jr., Dan Coates, Ellen Cohn, and Louise Kidder. 1982. Models of helping and coping. *American Psychologist* 37 (4): 368–384,

Brock, Leslie, and Eugene Aronowitz. 1982. The role of the self-help clearinghouse. In *Prevention in Human Services* 1 (3): 121–129.

Brody, Howard. 1987. *Stories of Sickness*. New Haven: Yale University Press.

Brown, Stephanie. 1993. Therapeutic process in Alcoholics Anonymous. In *Research on Alcoholics Anonymous: Opportunities and Alternatives*, edited by Barbara S. McCrady and William R. Miller. New Brunswick, N.J.: Rutgers Center of Alcohol Studies.

Bruner, Jerome. 1986. *Actual Minds, Possible Worlds*. Cambridge, Mass.: Harvard University Press.

———. 1990. *Acts of Meaning*. Cambridge, Mass.: Harvard University Press.

Bucher, Rue. 1962. Pathology: A study of social movements within the profession. *Social Problems* 10 (Summer): 40–51.

Bufe, Charles. 1991. *Alcoholics Anonymous: Cult or Cure*. San Francisco: Sharp Press.

Caetano, Raul. 1993. Ethnic minority groups and Alcoholics Anonymous: A review. In *Research on Alcoholics Anonymous: Opportunities and Alternatives*, edited by Barbara S. McGrady and William R. Miller. New Brunswick, N.J.: Rutgers Center of Alcohol Studies.

Cain, Carole. 1991. Personal stories: Identity acquisition and self-understanding in Alcoholics Anonymous. *Ethos* 19 (2): 210–251.

Campbell, James. 1995. *Understanding John Dewey: Nature and Cooperative Intelligence*. Chicago: Open Court Publishing Co.

Caplan, Gerald, and Marie Killilea, eds. 1976. *Support Systems and Mutual Help: Multidisciplinary Explorations*. New York: Grune and Stratton.

Capra, F. 1996. *The Web of Life*. New York: Anchor.

Carroll, Stephanie. 1993. Spirituality and purpose in life in alcoholism recovery. *Journal of Studies on Alcohol* (May): 297–301.

Cavanaugh, Christopher. 1998. *AA to Z: Addictionary to the 12-Step Culture*. New York: Main Street Books Doubleday.

Checkoway, Barry, Mark Chesler, and Stephen Blum. 1990. Self-care, self-help, and community care for health. In *Working with Self-Help*, edited by Thomas Powell. Silver Spring, Md.: National Association of Social Workers Press.

Chesler, Mark A. 1990. The "dangers" of self-help groups: Understanding and challenging professionals' views. In *Working with Self-Help*, edited by Thomas Powell. Silver Spring, Md.: National Association of Social Workers Press.

———. 1991. Participatory action research with self-help groups: An alternative paradigm for inquiry and action. *American Journal of Community Psychology* 19 (5): 757–768.

Chesler, Mark A., and Barbara K. Chesney. 1995. *Cancer and Self-Help: Bridging the Troubled Waters of Childhood Illness*. Madison: University of Wisconsin Press.

Chesler, Mark A., Barbara Chesney, and Benjamin Gidron. 1990. Israeli and U.S. orientations toward self-help groups for families in crisis. *Nonprofit and Voluntary Sector Quarterly* 19 (3): 251–262.

Chesler, Mark A. and Margaret Yoak. 1984. Self-help groups for parents of children with cancer. In *Helping Patients and Their Families Cope with Medical Problems*, edited by Howard Roback. San Francisco: Jossey-Bass.

Church, Kathryn. 1996. Beyond "bad manners": The power relations of "consumer participation" in Ontario's community mental health system. *Canadian Journal of Community Mental Health* 15 (2): 27–44.

Cockerham, William. 1998. *Medical Sociology.* 7th ed. Upper Saddle River, N.J.: Prentice Hall.

Coleman, James. 1990. *Foundations of Social Theory.* Cambridge, Mass.: Belknap Press of Harvard University Press.

Collins, Patricia Hill. 1993. Black feminist thought in the matrix of domination. In *Social Theory: The Multicultural and Classic Readings,* edited by Charles Lemert. Boulder, Colo.: Westview Press.

Conrad, Peter, and Joseph W. Schneider. 1980. *Deviance and Medicalization: From Badness to Sickness.* St. Louis: C. V. Mosby.

Cook, Scott D., and Dvora Yanow. 1993. Culture and organizational learning. *Journal of Management Inquiry* 2 (4): 373–390.

Coyle, Sandra. 1996. Restructuring self: Using deep learning groups among Adult Children of Alcoholics. *Clinical Sociology Review* 14: 103–118.

Crawford, Shea E. 1997. Rational-legal authority and experiential authority in social model programs. M.A. thesis, George Mason University, Fairfax, Va.

Cross, Patricia K. 1988. *Adults as Learners.* San Francisco: Jossey-Bass.

Cummings, Michael, Marshall H. Becker, and Marla C. Maile. 1980. Bringing the models together: An empirical approach to combining variables used to explain health actions. *Journal of Behavioral Medicine* 3 (2): 123–145.

D'Asaro, Andrea. 1994. Connecting with computer bulletin boards. *The Key.* National Mental Health Consumers' Self-Help Clearinghouse Newsletter. 2 (2): 1–8.

Davidson, Larry, Matthew Chinman, Bret Kloos, Richard Weingarten, David Stayner, and Jacob Kraemer Tebes. 1997. Peer support among individuals with severe mental illness: History, roadblocks, and a review of the evidence. Paper prepared for the Self-Help Research Pre-Conference, Society for Community Research and Action Biennial Conference, May 28, Greensboro, S.C.

Davison, Gerald C., and John M. Neale. 1998. *Abnormal Psychology.* 7th ed. New York: John Wiley and Sons.

Denzin, Norman, and Yvonne Lincoln. 1994. *Handbook of Qualitative Research.* Newbury Park, Calif.: Sage.

Dewey, John. 1938. *Experience and Education.* New York: Collier Books, Macmillan Publishing.

Dicke, Lisa, and J. Steven Ott. 1997. Public agency accountability in human services contracting. Paper presented at the 26th annual conference of ARNOVA, December 4, Indianapolis, Ind.

DiClemente, Carlos. 1993. Alcoholics Anonymous and the structure of change. In *Research on Alcoholics Anonymous: Opportunities and Alternatives,* edited by Barbara McCrady and William R. Miller. New Brunswick, N.J.: Rutgers Center of Alcohol Studies.

Dixon, Nancy. 1994. *The Organizational Learning Cycle: How We Can Learn Collectively.* London: McGraw-Hill.

DuPont, Robert, and John P. McGovern. 1994. *A Bridge to Recovery: An Introduction to 12-Step Programs.* Washington, D.C.: American Psychiatric Press.

Edmunson, E. D., J. R. Bedell, et al. 1982. Integrating skill building and peer support in mental health treatment: The early intervention and community network development projects. In *Community Mental Health and Behavioral Ecology: A Handbook of Theory, Research, and Practice,* edited by Abraham M. Jeger and Robert S. Slotnick. New York: Plenum Press.

Emerick, Robert E. 1989. Group demographics in the mental patient movement: Group location, age, and size as structural factors. *Community Mental Health Journal* 25 (4): 277–299.

———. 1991. The politics of psychiatric self-help: Political factors, interactional support, and group longevity in a social movement. *Social Science and Medicine* 32 (10): 1121–1128.

———. 1996. Mad liberation: The sociology of knowledge and the ultimate civil rights movement. *Journal of Mind and Behavior* 17 (2): 135–160.

Emery, F. E., and E. L. Trist. 1965. The causal texture of organizational environments. *Human Relations* 18: 21–32.

Etzioni, Amitai. 1964. *Modern Organizations*. Englewood Cliffs, N.J.: Prentice Hall.

Farquharson, Andy. 1995. Developing a self-help perspective: Conversations with professionals. *Canadian Journal of Community Mental Health* 14, 2 (Fall): 81–89.

Forsyth, Donelson R. 1990. *Group Dynamics*. 2nd ed. Pacific Grove, Calif.: Brooks/ Cole Publishing.

Fowler, James W. 1993. Alcoholics Anonymous and faith development. In *Research on Alcoholics Anonymous: Opportunities and Alternatives*, edited by Barbara S. McCrady and William R. Miller. New Brunswick, N.J.: Rutgers Center of Alcohol Studies.

Fox, Renee C. 1986. The medicalization and demedicalization of American society. In *The Sociology of Health and Illness: Critical Perspectives*. 2nd ed. Edited by Peter Conrad and Rochelle Kern. New York: St. Martin's Press.

Franklin, Mary Beth. 1998. Researching your own disease. *The Washington Post*, August 4, Health Section, 10–13.

Freire, Paulo. 1970. *Pedagogy of the Oppressed*. New York: Seabury Press.

Friedson, Eliot. 1970a. *Profession of Medicine*. New York: Dodd and Mead.

———. 1970b. *Professional Dominance*. Chicago: Aldine.

———, ed. 1973. *The Professions and Their Prospects*. Beverly Hills, Calif.: Sage Publications.

Gartner, Alan, and Frank Riessman. 1977. *Self-Help in the Human Services*. San Francisco: Jossey-Bass.

Gartner, Audrey J. 1997. Professionals and self-help: Can they get along? *Social Policy* 27 (Spring): 47–52.

Gellman, Irving P. 1964. *The Sober Alcoholic: An Organizational Analysis of Alcoholics Anonymous*. New Haven, Conn.: College and University Press.

Gibson, James J. 1979. *The Ecological Approach to Visual Perception*. Boston: Houghton Mifflin.

Giddens, Anthony. 1990. *The Consequences of Modernity*. Stanford: Stanford University Press.

———. 1993. Post-modernity or radicalised modernity? In *Social Theory: The Multicultural and Classic Readings*, edited by Charles Lemert. Boulder, Colo.: Westview Press.

Gidron, Benjamin, and Mark Chesler. 1994. Universal and particular attributes of self-help: A framework for international and intranational analysis. In *Self-Help and Mutual Aid Groups: International and Multicultural Perspectives*, edited by Francine Lavoie, Thomasina Borkman, and Benjamin Gidron. New York: Haworth Press.

Gleick, James. 1987. *Chaos: Making a New Science*. New York: Viking Press.

Goffman, Erving. 1963. *Stigma: Notes on the Management of Spoiled Identity*. Englewood Cliffs, N.J.: Prentice Hall.

Gold, Gerald. 1995. Chronic illness and disability in an electronic support group. Paper presented at the annual meeting of the Society for Applied Anthropology, March 31, Albuquerque, N.M.

Goldberger, Nancy Rule. 1996. Introduction: Looking backward, looking forward." In *Knowledge, Difference, and Power: Essays Inspired by Women's Ways of Knowing*, edited by Nancy Rule Goldberger, Jill Mattuck Tarule, Blythe McVicker Clinchy, and Mary Field Belenky. New York: Basic Books.

Goldberger, Nancy Rule, Jill Mattuck Tarule, Blythe McVicker Clinchy, and Mary Field Belenky, eds. 1996. *Knowledge, Difference and Power: Essays Inspired by Women's Ways of Knowing*. New York: Basic Books.

Goldstein, J. 1994. *The Unshackled Organization*. Portland, Ore.: Productivity Press.

Goode, Erich. 1997. *Deviant Behavior*. 5th ed. Upper Saddle River, N.J.: Prentice Hall.

Gottlieb, Benjamin, and Larry Peters. 1991. A national demographic portrait of mutual aid group participants in Canada. *American Journal of Community Psychology* 19 (5): 651–666.

Gottlieb, Naomi. 1992. Empowerment, political analyses, and services for women. In *Human Services as Complex Organizations*, edited by Yeheskel Hasenfeld. Newbury Park, Calif.: Sage Publications.

Gouldner, Alvin W. 1993. Toward a reflexive sociology. In *Social Theory: The Multicultural and Classic Readings*, edited by Charles Lemert. Boulder, Colo.: Westview Press.

Grandin, Temple. 1995. *Thinking in Pictures: And Other Reports from My Life with Autism*. New York: Vintage Books.

Gray, Bradford, H. 1991. *The Profit Motive and Patient Care: The Changing Accountability of Doctors and Hospitals*. Cambridge, Mass.: Harvard University Press.

Gronbjerg, Kirsten A. 1992. Nonprofit human service organizations: Funding strategies and patterns of adaptation. In *Human Services as Complex Organizations*, edited by Yeheskel Hasenfeld. Newbury Park, Calif.: Sage Publications.

Habermas, Jürgen. 1971. *Knowledge and Human Interests*. Boston: Beacon Press.

——. 1981. New social movements. *Telos*, no. 49: 33–37.

Hager, Mark. 1997. Neither adaptation nor selection: "Mission completion" as a rationale for organizational dissolution. Paper presented at the 26th annual conference of ARNOVA, 4–6 December, Indianapolis, Ind.

Hall, Richard. 1996. *Organizations: Structures, Processes, and Outcomes*. 6th ed. Englewood Cliffs, N.J.: Prentice Hall.

Hannah, Michael T., and John Freeman. 1977. The population ecology of organizations. *American Journal of Sociology* 82: 929–964.

——. 1989. *Organizational Ecology*. Cambridge, Mass.: Harvard University Press.

Harding, Sandra. 1991. *Whose Science? Whose Knowledge? Thinking from Women's Lives*. Ithaca, N.Y.: Cornell University Press.

——. 1996. Gendered ways of knowing and the "epistemological crisis" of the West. In *Knowledge, Difference, and Power: Essays Inspired by Women's Ways of Knowing*, edited by Nancy Rule Goldberger, Jill Mattuck Tarule, Blythe McVicker Clinchy, and Mary Field Belenky. New York: Basic Books.

Hasenfeld, Yeheskel. 1972. People processing organizations: An exchange approach. *American Sociological Review* 37: 256–263.

Hasenfeld, Yeheskel, and Benjamin Gidron. 1993. Self-help groups and human service organizations: An interorganizational perspective. *Social Service Review* 2: 217–235.

Hatfield, Agnes B., and Harriet P. Lefley. 1993. *Surviving Mental Illness: Stress, Coping, and Adaptation*. New York: Guilford Press.

Hedrick, Hannah, Daryl Isenberg, and C. Martini. 1992. Self-help groups: Empowerment through policy and partnerships. In *Self-Help: Concepts and Applications*, edited by Alfred Katz, Hannah L. Hedrick, Daryl Holtz Isenberg, Leslie M. Thompson, Therese Goodrich, and Austin H. Kutscher. Philadelphia: Charles Press.

Helgesen, Sally. 1998. *Everyday Revolutionaries: Working Women and the Transformation of American Life*. New York: Doubleday.

Hicks, Frances, and Thomasina Borkman. 1988. Self-help groups and political empowerment. Paper presented at the annual meeting of the American Political Science Association, September 3, Washington, D.C.

Hodgkinson, Virginia A., Richard W. Lyman, and associates, eds. 1989. *The Future of the Nonprofit Sector: Challenges, Changes, and Policy Considerations*. San Francisco: Jossey-Bass.

Howes, Joanne, and Amy Allina. 1994. Women's health movements. *Social Policy* 24 (4): 6–14.

Hughes, Robert. 1993. *The Culture of Complaint: The Fraying of America*. New York: Oxford University Press.

Humphreys, Keith. 1997. Individual and social benefits of mutual aid/self-help groups. *Social Policy* (Spring): 12–19.

Humphreys, Keith, and Jennifer M. Noke. 1997. The influence of post-treatment mutual help group participation on the friendship networks of substance abuse patients. *American Journal of Community Psychology* 25 (1): 1–16.

Humphreys, Keith, B. Mavis, and B. Stoffelmayr. 1994. Are twelve step programs appropriate for disenfranchised groups? Evidence from a study of post-treatment mutual help involvement. In *Self-Help and Mutual Aid Groups: International and Multicultural Perspectives*, edited by Francine Lavoie, Thomasina Borkman, and Benjamin Gidron. New York: Haworth Press.

Humphreys, Keith, and Julian Rappaport. 1994. Researching self-help/mutual aid groups and organizations: Many roads, one journey. *Applied and Preventive Psychology* 3: 217–231.

Humphreys, Keith, and Michael D. Woods. 1994. Researching mutual help group affiliation in a segregated society. In *Understanding Self-Help Organizations: Frameworks and Findings*, edited by Thomas J. Powell. Thousand Oaks, Calif.: Sage.

Hurvitz, Nathan. 1976. The origins of the peer self-help psychotherapy group movement. In the Special Issue on Self-Help Groups, *Journal of Applied Behavioral Science* 12 (3): 283–294.

Iannello, Kathleen P. 1992. *Decisions without Hierarchy: Feminist Interventions in Organization Theory and Practice*. New York: Routledge.

Jacobs, Marion K., and Gerald Goodman. 1989. Psychology and self-help groups: Predictions on a partnership. *American Psychologist* 44: 1–10.

James, William. 1978. *The Varieties of Religious Experience*. Garden City, N.Y.: Image Books.

Janz, Nancy, and Marshall Becker. 1984. The health belief model: A decade later. *Health Education Quarterly* 11 (1): 1–47.

Jemmott, Frances E. 1997. Self-help and philanthropy: Ready or not, here they come. *Social Policy* 27 (3): 53–55.

Jenkins, Richard, and Kenneth I. Pargamet. 1995. Religion and spirituality as resources for coping with cancer. *Journal of Psychosocial Oncology* 13 (1/2): 51–74.

Jezer, Marty. 1997. *Stuttering: A Life Bound Up in Words*. New York: Basic Books.

Johnson, David W., and Frank P. Johnson. 1997. *Joining Together: Group Therapy and Group Skills*. Boston: Allyn and Bacon.

Kallick, David D. 1949. New frameworks for health-care reform. *Social Policy* 24 (spring): 2–5.

Kaminer, Wendy. 1993. *I'm Dysfunctional, You're Dysfunctional: The Recovery Movement and Other Self-Help Fashions*. New York: Vintage.

Kanter, Rosabeth Moss. 1972. *Commitment and Community: Communes and Utopias in Sociological Perspective*. Cambridge, Mass.: Harvard University Press.

Kaskutas, Lee Ann. 1992. Beliefs on the source of sobriety: Interactions of membership in Women for Sobriety and Alcoholics Anonymous. *Contemporary Drug Problems* (Winter): 631–648.

———. 1994. What do women get out of self-help? Their reasons for attending Women for Sobriety and Alcoholics Anonymous. *Journal of Substance Abuse Treatment* 11 (3): 185–195.

———. 1995. Personal correspondence with author.

———. 1998. Hip and helpful: Alcoholics Anonymous in Marin County, California. In *Diversity in Unity: Studies of Alcoholics Anonymous in Eight Societies*, edited by Pia Rosenqvist and Irmgard Eisenbach-Stengl. Helsinki: Nordic Council for Alcohol and Drug Research.

Kaskutas, Lee Ann, Deborah Marsh, and Abigail Kohn. 1998. Didactic and experiential education in substance abuse programs. *Journal of Substance Abuse Treatment* 15 (1): 43–53.

Kaskutas, Lee Ann, and Thomas A. McLellan, eds. 1998. The social model approach to substance abuse recovery. *Journal of Substance Abuse Treatment* 15 (1): 1–85.

Kasl, Charlotte Davis. 1992. *Many Roads, One Journey: Moving Beyond the Twelve Steps*. New York: Harper Perennial.

Katz, Alfred H. 1961. *Parents of the Handicapped*. Springfield, Ill.: Charles C. Thomas.

———. 1993. *Self-Help Groups as Social Movement*. Oakland: Twane Publishers.

Katz, Alfred H., and Eugene I. Bender. 1976. Self-help groups in Western society: History and prospects. *Journal of Applied Behavioral Science* 12 (3): 265–282.

———, eds. 1990. *Helping One Another: Self-Help Groups in a Changing World*. Oakland, Calif.: Third Party Publishing.

Katz, Alfred H., Hannah L. Hedrick, Daryl Holtz Isenberg, Leslie M. Thompson, Therese Goodrich, and Austin H. Kutscher, eds. 1992. *Self-Help: Concepts and Applications*. Philadelphia: Charles Press.

Katz, Alfred H., and Aimee E. Liu. 1991. *The Codependency Conspiracy: How to Break the Recovery Habit and Take Charge of Your Life*. New York: Warner Books.

Katz, Alfred H., and Carl A. Maida. 1990. Health and disability self-help organizations. In *Working with Self-Help*, edited by Thomas J. Powell. Silver Spring, Md.: National Association of Social Workers Press.

Kaufmann, Caroline L., Herbert Schulberg, and Nina Schooler. 1994. Self-help group participation among people with severe mental illness. In *Self-Help and Mutual Aid Groups: International and Multicultural Perspectives*, edited by Francine Lavoie, Thomasina Borkman, and Benjamin Gidron. New York: Haworth Press.

Kennedy, Mellen. 1990. Psychiatric hospitalization of GROWers. Paper presented at the Second Biennial Conference on Community Research and Action, East Lansing, Mich.

Kennedy, Mellen, and Keith Humphreys. 1994. Understanding worldview transformation in members of mutual help groups. *Prevention in Human Services* 11 (1): 181–198.

Kennedy, S., J. K. Kiecolt-Glaser, and R. Glaser. 1988. Immunological consequences of acute and chronic stressors: Mediating role of interpersonal relationships. *British Journal of Medical Psychology* 61: 77–85.

Kessler, Ronald C., Kristin D. Mickleson, and Shanyang Zhao. 1997. Patterns and correlates of self-help group membership in the United States. *Social Policy* 27 (3): 27–46.

Kiecolt-Glaser, J. K., J. T. Cacioppo, W. B. Malarkey, and R. Glaser. 1992. Acute psychological stressors and short-term immune changes: What, why, for whom, and to what extent? *Psychosomatic Medicine* 54: 680–685.

Kiecolt-Glaser, J. K., and R. Glaser. 1995. Psychoneuroimmunology and health consequences: Data and shared mechanisms. *Psychosomatic Medicine* 57: 269–274.

Kiecolt-Glaser, J. K., P. T. Marucha, W. B. Malarkey, A. M. Mercado, and R. Glaser. 1995. Slowing of wound healing by psychological stress. *Lancet* 346: 1194–1196.

Killilea, Marie. 1976. Mutual help organizations: Interpretations in the literature. In *Support Systems and Mutual Help: Multidisciplinary Explorations*, edited by Gerald Kaplan and Marie Killilea. New York: Grune and Stratton.

Kleist, Jeffrey. 1990. Network resource utilization patterns of members of Alcoholics Anonymous. Ph.D. diss., University of Akron, Ohio.

Kolb, David. 1984. *Experiential Learning: Experience as the Source of Learning and Development*. Englewood Cliffs, N.J.: Prentice Hall.

Kropotkin, Petr. [1914] 1972. *Mutual Aid: A Factor in Evolution*. New York: New York University Press.

Kurtz, Ernest. 1979. *Not-God: A History of Alcoholics Anonymous*. Center City, Minn.: Hazelden.

———. 1981. Why A.A. works: The intellectual significance of AA. *Journal of Studies on Alcohol* 43 (1): 38–80.

Kurtz, Ernest, and Katherine Ketcham. 1992. *The Spirituality of Imperfection: Modern Wisdom from Classic Stories*. New York: Bantam Books.

Kurtz, Linda Farris. 1988. Mutual aid for affective disorders: the manic depressive and depressive association. *American Journal of Orthopsychiatry* 58 (1): 152–155.

———. 1997. *Self-Help and Support Groups: A Handbook for Practitioners*. Thousand Oaks, Calif.: Sage.

Lakoff, George, and Mark Johnson. 1980. *Metaphors We Live By*. Chicago: University of Chicago Press.

Lavoie, Francine, Andy Farquharson, and Mellen Kennedy. 1994. Workshop on "good practice" in the collaboration between professionals and mutual aid groups. In *Prevention in Human Services* 11 (2): 303–314.

Lavoie, Francine, Thomasina Borkman, and Benjamin Gidron, eds. 1994. *Self-Help and Mutual Aid Groups: International and Multicultural Perspectives*. New York: Haworth Press.

Lefton, Mark, and William Rosengren. 1966. Organizations and clients: Lateral and longitudinal dimensions. *American Sociological Review* 31 (December): 802–810.

Lemert, Charles, ed. 1993. *Social Theory: The Multicultural and Classic Readings*. Boulder, Colo.: Westview Press.

Lemert, Edwin M. 1951. *Social Pathology*. New York: McGraw-Hill.

Lenrow, Peter, and Rosemary Burch. 1981. Mutual aid or professional services: Opposing or complementary? In *Social Network and Social Support*, edited by Benjamin Gottlieb. Beverly Hills, Calif.: Sage.

Let's Face It. 1997. *Resources for People with Facial Difference*. Bellingham, Wash.: Let's Face It.

Levy, Leon. 1976. Self-help groups: Types and psychological processes. *Journal of Applied Behavioral Science* 12: 310–322.

Levy, Leon, and J. F. Derby. 1992. Bereavement support groups: Who joins, who does not, and why. *Journal of Community Psychology* 20: 649–662.

Lieberman, Morton A., and Leonard I. Borman. 1976. Introduction to the Special Issue on Self-Help Groups. *Journal of Applied Behavioral Science* 12 (3): 261–264.

Lieberman, Morton A., and Lonnie R. Snowden. 1993. Problems in assessing prevalence and membership characteristics of self-help group participants. *Journal of Applied Behavioral Science* 29, 2: 166–180.

Lofland, John. 1969. *Deviance and Identity*. Englewood Cliffs, N.J.: Prentice Hall.

Lohmann, Roger A. 1992. *The Commons: New Perspectives on Nonprofit Organizations and Voluntary Action*. San Francisco: Jossey-Bass.

Long, Douglas G. 1990. *Learner Managed Learning: The Key to Lifelong Learning and Development*. New York: St. Martin's Press.

Low, Abraham. 1950. *Mental Health through Will Training*. Chicago: Willett Publishing.

Luke, Douglas A., Linda Roberts, and Julian Rappaport. 1993. Individual, group context, and individual-group fit predictors of self-help group attendance. *Journal of Applied Behavioral Science* 29 (2): 216–238.

Lupton, Deborah. 1994. *Medicine as Culture: Illness, Disease, and the Body in Western Societies*. Thousand Oaks, Calif.: Sage.

Lyotard, Jean-François. 1993. The postmodern condition. In *Social Theory: The Multicultural and Classic Readings*, edited by Charles Lemert. Boulder, Colo.: Westview Press.

Madara, Edward J. 1986. A comprehensive systems approach to promoting mutual aid self-help groups: The New Jersey Clearinghouse model. *Journal of Voluntary Action Research* 15 (2): 57–63.

———. 1992. The primary value of a self-help clearinghouse. In *Self-Help: Concepts and Applications*, edited by Alfred H. Katz, Hannah L. Hedrick, Daryl Holtz Isenberg, Leslie M. Thompson, Therese Goodrich, and Austin H. Kutscher. Philadelphia: Charles Press.

———. 1995. Personal communication with author.

———. 1997. The mutual-aid self-help online revolution. *Social Policy* 27 (3): 20–26.

———. 1998. Developing self-help groups: Ten steps and suggestions for professionals. In *The Self-Help Sourcebook: Your Guide to Community and Online Support Groups*. 6th ed. Edited by Barbara J. White and Edward J. Madara. Denville, N.J.: Northwest Covenant Medical Center.

Madara, Edward J., John Kalafat, and Bruce Miller. 1988. The computerized self-help clearinghouse: Using "high tech" to promote "high touch" support networks. *Computers in Human Services* 3 (3/4): 39–52.

Maida, Carl, Alfred H. Katz, Gayle Strauss, and Cecelia Kwa. 1992. Self-help, social networks, and social adaptation in lupus. In *Self-Help: Concepts and Applications*, edited by Alfred Katz, Hannah Hedrick, Daryl Holtz Isenberg, Leslie M. Thompson, Therese Goodrich, and Austin H. Kutscher. Philadelphia: Charles Press.

Maier, Steven F., Linda Watkins, and Monika Fleshner. 1994. Psychoneuroimmunology: The interface between behavior, brain, and immunity. *American Psychologist* 49 (12): 1004–1017.

Makela, Klaus. 1993. Implications for research of the cultural variability of Alcoholics Anonymous. In *Research on Alcoholics Anonymous: Opportunities and Alternatives*, edited by Barbara S. McGrady and William R. Miller. New Brunswick, N.J.: Rutgers Center of Alcohol Studies.

Makela, Klaus, et al. 1996. *Alcoholics Anonymous as a Mutual-Help Movement: A Study in Eight Societies*. Madison: University of Wisconsin Press.

Mason, David E. 1996. *Leading and Managing the Expressive Dimension*. San Francisco: Jossey-Bass.

Maton, Kenneth I. 1993. Moving beyond the individual level of analysis in mutual help group research: An ecological paradigm. *Journal of Applied Behavioral Science* 29 (2): 272–286.

Mattingly, Cheryl. 1991. Narrative reflections on practical actions: Two learning experiences in reflective storytelling. In *The Reflective Turn: Case Studies in and on Educational Practice*, edited by Donald Schon. New York: Teachers College, Columbia University.

Maxwell, Milton A. 1984. *The AA Experience: A Close-Up View for Professionals*. New York: McGraw-Hill.

McCarthy, John, and Mayer Zald. 1977. Resource mobilization and social movements. *American Journal of Sociology* 82: 1212–1241.

McCowan, Joe. 1978. *Availability: Gabriel Marcel and the Phenomenology of Human Openness*. Missoula, Mt.: Scholars Press.

McGrady, Barbara, and William R. Miller. 1993. *Research on Alcoholics Anonymous: Opportunities and Alternatives*. New Brunswick, N.J.: Rutgers Center of Alcohol Studies.

McIntosh, Peggy. 1983. Interactive phases of curricular re-vision: A feminist perspective. Wellesley, Mass.: Wellesley College Center for Research on Women. Working Paper no. 124.

———. 1990. Interactive phases of curricular and personal revision with regard to race. Wellesley, Mass.: Center for Research on Women, Wellesley College. Working Paper no. 219.

McKinlay, John B., and Sonja M. McKinlay. 1994. Medical measures and the decline of mortality. In *The Sociology of Health and Illness: Critical Perspectives*, edited by Peter Conrad and Rochelle Kern, 4th ed. New York: St. Martin's Press.

McKnight, John. 1994. Politicizing health care. In *The Sociology of Health and Illness: Critical Perspectives*, edited by Peter Conrad and Rochelle Kern, 4th ed. New York: St. Martin's Press.

———. 1995. *The Careless Community: Community and Its Counterfeits*. New York: Basic Books.

Mead, George Herbert. [1934] 1962. *Mind, Self, and Society: From the Standpoint of a Social Behaviorist*, edited by Charles Morris. Chicago: University of Chicago Press.

Mead, Margaret. 1970. *Culture and Commitment: A Study of the Generation Gap*. New York: Columbia University Press.

Medvene, Louis, J. 1984. Self-help and professional collaboration. *Social Policy* 14 (Spring): 15–18.

Medvene, Louis, and David Krauss. 1985. An exploratory case study of the Hamden Connecticut chapter of Families of the Mentally Ill (FOMI). Yale University.

Medvene, Louis J., Keh-Ming Lin, Anges Wu, Richard Mendoza, Norma Harris, and Milton Miller. 1994. Mexican American and Anglo-American parents of the mentally ill: Attitudes and participation in family support groups. In *Self-Help and Mutual Aid Groups: International and Multicultural Perspectives*, edited by Francine Lavoie, Thomasina Borkman, and Benjamin Gidron. New York: Haworth Press.

Medvene, Louis J., Scott Wituk, and Douglas Luke. In press. Characteristics of self-help group leaders: The significance of professional and founder statuses. *International Journal of Self-Help and Self-Care* 1 (1): 101–115.

Meissen, Greg, and Mary Warren. 1997. Self-help groups and managed care: Building a research and action agenda. Paper prepared for the Self-Help Research Pre-Conference of the Society for Community Research and Action Biennial Conference, May 28, Greensboro, S.C.

Melucci, Alberto. 1985. The symbolic challenge of contemporary movements. *Social Research* 52 (Winter): 789–816.

Merriam, S. B., and R. S. Caffarella. 1991. *Learning in Adulthood*. San Francisco: Jossey-Bass.

Messer, John G. 1994. Emergent organization as a practical strategy: Executing trustee functions in Alcoholics Anonymous. *Nonprofit and Voluntary Sector Quarterly* 23 (4): 293–307.

Messer, John, and Thomasina Borkman. 1996. Functions and limits of private and public benefit in creating social capital: The role of self-help mutual aid in building community capacity. Paper presented at the 25th ARNOVA conference, November 7–9, New York.

Mestrovic, Stjepan. 1997. *Postemotional Society*. London: Sage.

Mezirow, Jack. 1991. *Transformative Dimensions of Adult Learning*. San Francisco: Jossey-Bass.

Michels, Robert. [1911] 1949. *Political Parties*. New York: Free Press.

Miller, Lenore. 1988. What health professionals can learn from breast cancer patients. In *Surgeon General's Workshop on Self-Help and Public Health*. U.S. Department of Health and Human Services, Public Health Resources, Health Resources and Services Administration, Bureau of Maternal Health and Child Health and Resources Development Publication no. 224–250. Washington, D.C.: U.S. Government Printing Office.

Miller, William, and Ernest Kurtz. 1994. Models of alcoholism used in treatment: Contrasting AA and other perspectives with which it is often confused. *Journal of Studies on Alcohol* (March): 159–166.

Milofsky, Carl. 1987. Neighborhood-based organizations: A market analogy. In *The Nonprofit Sector: A Research Handbook*, edited by Walter W. Powell. New Haven: Yale University Press.

———. 1988. Scarcity and community: A resource allocation theory of community and mass society organizations. In *Community Organizations: Studies in Resource Mobilization and Exchange*, edited by Carl Milofsky. New York: Oxford University Press.

Mitroff, Ian. 1998. *Smart Thinking for Crazy Times*. San Francisco: Berett-Koehler Publishers.

Moos, Rudolph H. 1974. *Evaluating Treatment Environments: A Social Ecological Approach*. New York: John Wiley.

Moos, Rudolph H., John Finney, and Peg Maude-Griffon. 1993. The social climate of self-help and mutual support groups: Assessing group implementation, process, and outcome. In *Research on Alcoholics Anonymous: Opportunities and Alternatives*, edited by Barbara S. McCrady and William R. Miller. New Brunswick, N.J.: Rutgers Center for Alcohol Studies.

Morgan, Gareth. 1986. *Images of Organization*. Newbury Park, Calif.: Sage Publications.

———. 1997. *Images of Organizations*. Thousand Oaks, Calif.: Sage.

Mullins, Fitzhugh. 1992. Rewriting the social contract in health. In *Self-Help: Concepts and Applications*, edited by Alfred Katz, Hannah L. Hedrick, Daryl Holtz Isenberg, Leslie M. Thompson, Therese Goodrich, and Austin H. Kutscher. Philadelphia: Charles Press.

Mumford, Emily. 1983. *Medical Sociology: Patients, Providers, and Policies*. New York: Random House.

Murphy, Robert F. 1990. *The Body Silent*. New York: W. W. Norton.

Neighbors, H. W., K. A. Elliott, and L. M. Gant. 1990. Self-help and Black Americans: A strategy for empowerment. In *Working with Self-Help*, edited by Thomas J. Powell. Silver Spring, Md.: National Association of Social Workers Press.

Nelson, Geoffrey. 1994. The development of a mental health coalition: A case study. *American Journal of Community Psychology* 22: 229–255.

Nussbaum, Bruce. 1990. *Good Intentions: How Big Business and the Medical Establishment Are Corrupting the Fight Against AIDS*. New York: Atlantic Monthly Press.

O'Leary, A. 1990. Stress, emotion, and human immune function. *Psychological Bulletin* 108: 363–382.

O'Neill, Michael. 1989. *The Third America: The Emergence of the Nonprofit Sector in the United States*. San Francisco: Jossey-Bass.

Oka, Tomofumi. 1994. Self-help groups in Japan: Trends and traditions. In *Self-Help and Mutual Aid Groups: International and Multicultural Perspectives*, edited by Francine Lavoie, Thomasina Borkman, and Benjamin Gidron. New York: Haworth Press.

Perkins, David V., Joan Esterline Lafuze, and Carole Van Dusen. 1994. Social climate correlates of effectiveness in Alliance for the Mentally Ill groups. *Self-Help and Mutual Aid Groups: International and Multicultural Perspectives*, edited by Francine Lavoie, Thomasina Borkman, and Benjamin Gidron. New York: Haworth Press.

Perrow, Charles. 1970. Members as resources in voluntary organizations. In *Organizations and Clients: Essays in the Sociology of Service*, edited by William R. Rosengren and Mark Lefton. Columbus, Ohio: Charles E. Merrill Publishing Company.

———. 1986. *Complex Organizations: A Critical Essay*. 3rd ed. New York: Random House.

Petersen, James C., and Gerald E. Markle. 1979a. The Laetrile controversy. In *Controversy: Politics of Technical Decisions*, edited by Dorothy Nelkin. Beverly Hills, Calif.: Sage Publications.

———. 1979b. Politics and science in the Laetrile controversy. In *Social Studies of Science*, vol. 9. Beverly Hills, Calif.: Sage Publications.

Petrunik, Michael. 1974. The quest for fluency: Fluency variations and the identity problems and management strategies of stutterers. In *Decency and Deviance*, edited by Jack Haas and William Shaffir. Toronto: McClelland and Stewart.

Phillips, Wende. 1996. A comparison of online, e-mail, and in-person self-help groups using Adult Children of Alcoholics as a model. <http://www.rider.edu/~suler/psycyber/acoa.html>

Polkinghorn, Donald. 1988. *Narrative Knowing and the Human Sciences*. Albany: State University of New York Press.

Pollner, Melvin, and Jill Stein. 1996. Narrative mapping of social worlds: The voice of experience in Alcoholics Anonymous. *Symbolic Interaction* 19 (3): 203–223.

Polyani, Michael. 1958. *Personal Knowledge: Towards a Post-Critical Philosophy*. Chicago: University of Chicago Press.

———. 1969. *Knowing and Being*. Chicago: University of Chicago Press.

Powell, Thomas J. 1987. *Self-Help Organizations and Professional Practice*. Silver Spring, Md.: National Association of Social Workers.

———. 1990. *Working with Self-Help*. Silver Spring, Md.: National Association of Social Workers.

———. 1994. Self-help research and policy issues. *Understanding the Self-Help Organization: Frameworks and Findings*. Thousand Oaks, Calif.: Sage Publications.

Powell, Walter, ed. 1987. *The Nonprofit Sector: A Research Handbook*. New Haven: Yale University Press.

Rappaport, Julian. 1993. Narrative studies, personal stories, and identity transformation in the mutual help context. *Journal of Applied Behavioral Science* 29 (2): 239–256.

Rappaport, Julian, E. Seidman, P. Toro, L. McFadden, T. Reischel, L. Roberts, D. Salem, and M. Zimmerman. 1985. Collaborative research with a mutual help organization. *Social Policy* 15 (3): 12–24.

Rapping, Elayne. 1997. There's self-help, and then there's self-help: Women in the recovery movement. *Social Policy* 27 (3): 56–61.

Reed, Edward S. 1996a. *Encountering the World: Toward a Ecological Psychology*. New York: Oxford University Press.

———. 1996b. *The Necessity of Experience*. New Haven: Yale University Press.

Remen, Rachel N. 1993. On defining spirit. *Noetic Sciences Review* 27: 41.

Remine, Daniel, Robert M. Rice, and Jenny Ross. 1984. *Self-Help Groups and Human Service Agencies: How They Work Together*. New York: Family Service of America.

Revenson, Tracey, and Brian J. Cassel. 1991. An exploration of leadership in a medical mutual help organization. *American Journal of Community Psychology* 19: 683–698.

Riches, Gordon, and Pam Dawson. 1996. Communities of feeling: The culture of bereaved parents. *Morality* 1 (2): 143–161.

Riessman, Frank. 1965. The "helper" therapy principle. *Social Work* 10 (2): 27–32.

———. 1982. The self-help ethos. *Social Policy* 12 (Summer): 42–43.

———. 1990a. Bashing self-help. *Self-Help Reporter* (Summer/Fall): 1–2.

———. 1990b. Restructuring help: A human services paradigm for the 1990's. *American Journal of Community Psychology*. 18, 2: 221–230.

Riessman, Frank, and David Carroll. 1995. *Redefining Self-Help: Policy and Practice*. San Francisco: Jossey-Bass.

Ritzer, George. 1993. *The McDonaldization of Society*. Thousand Oaks, Calif.: Pine Forge Press.

Robertson, Nan. 1988. *Getting Better: Inside Alcoholics Anonymous*. New York: William Morrow and Company.

Robinson, David, and Stuart Henry. 1977. *Self-Help and Health: Mutual Aid for Modern Problems*. London: Martin Robertson.

Rodin, Miriam. 1985. Getting on the program: A biocultural analysis of Alcoholics Anonymous. In *The American Experience with Alcohol: Contrasting Cultural Perspectives*, edited by L. A. Bennett and G. M. Ames. New York: Plenum Press.

Room, Robin. 1992. "Healing ourselves and our planet": The emergence and nature of a generalized twelve-step consciousness. *Contemporary Drug Problems* 19 (Winter): 717–740.

Room, Robin, and Thomas Greenfield. 1993. Alcoholics Anonymous, other 12–step movements, and psychotherapy in the U.S. general population, 1990. *Addiction* 88: 555–562.

Rosengren, William R., and Mark Lefton. 1969. *Hospitals and Patients*. New York: Atherton Press.

Rosenstock, Irwin. 1974. Historical origins of the health belief model. *Health Education Monographs* 2 (4): 328–335.

Rosovsky, Haydee, Leticia Casanova, Cuauhtemoc Perez-Lopez, and Arturo Naravez. 1992. Alcoholics Anonymous in Mexico. In *Drug Dependence: From the Molecular to the Social Level*, edited by Jaime Cohen-Yanez, Jose Luis Amezcua-Gastelum, Julian Villarreal, and Luis Salazar Zalava. Proceedings of the International Symposium on Drug Dependence: From the Molecular to the Social Level, January 22–25, Mexico City. Amsterdam: Elsevier.

Rudy, David R. 1986. *Becoming Alcoholic: Alcoholics Anonymous and the Reality of Alcoholism*. Carbondale: Southern Illinois University Press.

Sagarin, Edward. 1969. *Odd Man In: Societies of Deviants in America*. Chicago: Quadrangle Books.

Salamon, Lester M., and Helmut K. Anheier. 1994. *The Emerging Sector: An Overview*. Baltimore: Johns Hopkins University, Institute for Policy Studies.

Sarason, Seymour. 1972. *The Creation of Settings and the Future of Societies*. San Francisco: Jossey-Bass.

Sarbin, Theodore. 1986. The narrative as a root metaphor for psychology. In *Narrative Psychology: The Storied Nature of Human Conduct*, edited by T. Sarbin. New York: Praeger.

Scheler, Max. 1954. *The Nature of Sympathy*. Translated by Peter Heath. London: Routledge and Kegan Paul.

Schmitz, Kenneth L. 1986. The geography of the human person. *Communio* 13 (Spring): 27–48.

Schopler, Janice, and Maeda Galinsky. 1995. Expanding our view of support groups as open systems. In *Support Groups: Current Perspectives on Theory and Practice*, edited by M. Galinsky and J. Schopler. New York: Haworth Press.

Schubert, Marsha A. 1991. Investigating experiential knowledge in a self-help group. Ph.D. diss., George Mason University, Fairfax, Va.

Schubert, Marsha A., and Thomasina J. Borkman. 1991. An organizational typology for self-help groups. *American Journal of Community Psychology* 19 (5): 769–787.

———. 1994. Identifying the experiential knowledge created by a self-help group. In *Understanding Self-Help Organizations: Frameworks and Findings*, edited by Thomas Powell. Newbury Park, Calif.: Sage Publications.

Seabright, Mark A., and Jacques Delacroix. 1996. The minimalist organization as a postbureaucratic form: The example of Alcoholics Anonymous. *Journal of Management Inquiry* 5 (2): 140–154.

Self-Help Clearinghouse of Metropolitan Toronto, comp. 1994. *The Mutual Aid Guide. A Directory of Self-Help/Mutual Aid Groups in Metropolitan Toronto.*

Senge, Peter. 1990. *The Fifth Discipline: The Art and Practice of the Learning Organization.* New York: Doubleday.

Shaw, Sandra, and Thomasina J. Borkman, eds. 1990. *Social Model Alcohol Recovery: An Alternative to Traditional Clinical Treatment.* Burbank, Calif.: Bridge Focus.

Shaw, Richard, Mark Shaw, and Thomasina Borkman. 1985. Selected findings of a 1983 survey of self-help groups for persons who stutter. Report distributed to relevant national organizations.

Sheehan, Joseph G. 1965. Speech therapy and recovery from stuttering. *Journal of the California Speech and Hearing Association* 14: 3–7.

———. 1970. *Stuttering: Research and Therapy.* New York: Harper and Row.

Shivanandan, Mary. 1994. Interview by author. Bethesda, Md., June.

———. 1998. Interview by author. Bethesda, Md.

Silverman, Phyllis, and Diane Smith. 1984. "Helping" in mutual help groups for the physically disabled. In *The Self-Help Revolution*, edited by Frank Riessman and Alan Gartner. New York: Human Sciences Press.

Simon, Herbert A. 1991. Bounded rationality and organizational learning. *Organizational Science* 2: 125–134.

Smith, David Horton. 1994. Determinants of voluntary association participation and volunteering: A literature review. *Nonprofit and Voluntary Sector Quarterly* 23 (3): 243–263.

———. 1997a. The rest of the nonprofit sector: Grassroots associations as the dark matter ignored in prevailing "flat earth" maps of the sector. *Nonprofit and Voluntary Sector Quarterly* 26 (2): 114–131.

———. 1997b. Grassroots associations are important: Some theory and a review of the impact literature. *Nonprofit and Voluntary Sector Quarterly* 26 (3): 269–306.

Smith, Steven Rathgeb, and Michael Lipsky. 1993. *Nonprofits for Hire: The Welfare State in the Age of Contracting.* Cambridge, Mass.: Harvard University Press.

Snow, Matthew, James O. Prochaska, and Joseph Rossi. 1994. Processes of change in Alcoholics Anonymous: Maintenance factors in long-term sobriety. *Journal of Studies of Alcohol* 55: 362–371.

Spalding, Alison, and Gary J. Metz. 1997. Spirituality and quality of life in Alcoholics Anonymous. *Alcoholism Treatment Quarterly* 15 (1): 1–14.

Speigel, D., J. R. Bloom, H. C. Kraemer, and E. Gottheil. 1989. Effect of psychosocial treatment on survival of patients with metastatic breast cancer. *Lancet* (October): 888–891.

Stacey, Ralph D. 1992. *Managing the Unknowable: Strategic Boundaries between Order and Chaos in Organizations.* San Francisco: Jossey-Bass.

Starr, Paul. 1982. *The Social Transformation of American Medicine.* New York: Basic Books.

Straussner, Shulamith, Lala Ashenberg, and Betsy Robin Spiegel. 1996. An analysis of 12–step programs for substance abusers from a developmental perspective. *Clinical Social Work Journal* 24 (3): 299–309.

Steinberg, Mark, and Carrie Miles. 1979. Transformation of a group for the widowed. In *Self-Help Groups for Coping with Crisis*, edited by Morton A. Lieberman. San Francisco: Jossey-Bass.

Stevens, Rosemary. 1971. *American Medicine and the Public Interest.* New Haven, Conn.: Yale University Press.

Stewart, Miriam J. 1990a. Expanding theoretical conceptualizations of self-help groups. *Social Science and Medicine* 31 (9): 1057–1066.

Stewart, Miriam. 1990b. Professional interface with self-help mutual aid groups. *Social Science & Medicine* 31 (10): 1143–1158.

Stewart, Miriam, Sheila Banks, Douglas Crossman, and Dale Poel. 1994. Partnerships between health professionals and self-help groups: meanings and mechanisms. In *Self-Help and Mutual Aid Groups: International and Multicultural Perspectives*, edited by Francine Lavoie, Thomasina Borkman, and Benjamin Gidron. New York: Haworth Press.

Surgeon General Workshop on Self-Help and Public Health. 1988. U.S. Department of Health and Human Services, Public Health Services, Health Resources and Services Administration, Bureau of Maternal Health and Child Health and Resources Development Publication no. 224–250. Washington, D.C.: U.S. Government Printing Office.

Sutro, Livingston D. 1989. Alcoholics Anonymous in a Mexican peasant-indian village. *Human Organization* 48 (2): 180–186.

Tannen, Deborah. 1990. *You Just Don't Understand: Women and Men in Conversation.* New York: William Morrow and Company.

Taylor, Shelley E. 1995. *Health Psychology.* 3rd ed. New York: McGraw Hill.

Taylor, Shelley E., R. L. Falke, S. J. Shoptaw, and R. R. Lichtman. 1986. Social support, support groups, and the cancer patient. *Journal of Consulting and Clinical Psychology* 54: 608–615.

Thorpe, Mary, Richard Edwards, and Ann Hansons, eds. 1993. *Culture and Process of Adult Learning.* London: Routledge.

Todres, Rubin. 1982. Professional attitudes: Awareness and use of self-help groups. *Prevention in Human Services* 1: 91–98.

———. 1995. Self-help/mutual aid clearinghouses and groups in Canada: Recent developments. *Canadian Journal of Community Mental Health* 14 (2): 123–130.

Todres, Rubin, and Stephen Hagarty. 1993. An evaluation of a self-help clearinghouse: Awareness, knowledge, and utilization. *Canadian Journal of Community Mental Health* 12 (1): 211–223.

Toffler, Alvin. 1980. *The Third Wave.* New York: William and Murrow.

Touraine, A. 1985. An introduction to the study of social movements. *Social Research* 52: 749–787.

Trojan, Alf, Edith Halves, Hans-Wilhelm Wetendorf, and Rudolph Bauer. 1990. Activity areas and developmental stages in self-help groups. *Nonprofit and Voluntary Sector Quarterly* 19 (3): 263–278.

Tuijnman, Albert, and Max van der Kamp. 1992. *Learning across the Lifespan: Theories, Research, Policies*. Oxford: Pergamon Press.

Turnbull, Liz. 1997. Narcissism and the potential for self-transformation in the Twelve Steps. *Health* 1 (2): 149–165.

Turner, Bryan S. 1995. *Medical Power and Social Knowledge*. 2nd ed. London: Sage Publishers.

United States Census Bureau. 1975. *Historical Statistics of the United States: Colonial Times to 1970*. Bicentennial Edition. Washington, D.C.: U.S. Government Printing Office.

Van Riper, Charles. 1963. *Speech Correction: Principles and Methods*, 4th ed. Englewood Cliffs, N.J.: Prentice-Hall.

————. 1971. *The Nature of Stuttering*. Englewood Cliffs, N.J.: Prentice-Hall.

Vella, Jane. 1994. *Learning to Listen, Learning to Teach: The Power of Dialogue in Teaching Adults*. San Francisco: Jossey-Bass.

von Appen, Ursula. 1994. The development of self-help in Germany's new provinces (former East Germany): The case of Schwerin. In *Self-Help and Mutual Aid Groups: International and Multicultural Perspectives*. Edited by Francine Lavoie, Thomasina Borkman, and Benjamin Gidron. New York: Haworth Press.

Von Til, Jon. 1988. *Mapping the Third Sector: Voluntarism in a Changing Social Economy*. New York: Foundation Center.

Vourakis, Christine. 1989. The process of recovery for women in AA: Seeking groups like me. Ph.D. diss., School of Nursing, University of California, San Francisco.

Weber, George H. 1982. Self-help and beliefs. In *Beliefs and Self-Help*, edited by George H. Weber and Lucy Cohen. New York: Human Sciences Press.

Weber, Max. 1968. *Economy and Society: An Outline of Interpretive Sociology*. Translated by Ephraim Fischoff et al. Edited by Guenther Roth and Claus Wittich. New York: Bedminster Press.

Weick, Karl. 1991. The non-traditional quality of organizational learning. *Organizational Science* 2 (1): 116–124.

Weinberg, Nancy, John Schmale, Janet Uken, and Keith Wessel. 1996. Online help: Cancer patients participate in a computer-mediated support group. *Health and Social Work* 21 (1): 24–29.

Weisbrod, Burton A. 1988. *The Nonprofit Economy*. Cambridge, Mass.: Harvard University Press.

Weiss, Joan O., Jane Karkalits, Kathleen K. Bishop, and Natalie Paul, eds. 1986. *Genetics Support Groups: Volunteers and Professionals as Partners*. White Plains, N.Y.: March of Dimes Defects Foundation.

Wheatley, Margaret. 1992. *Leadership and the New Science*. San Francisco: Berrett-Koehler.

White, Barbara J., and Edward J. Madara, eds. 1998. *The Self-Help Sourcebook: Your Guide to Community and Online Support Groups*. 6th ed. Denville, N.J.: Northwest Covenant Medical Center.

Willen, Mildred. 1984. Parents Anonymous: The professional's role as sponsor. In *The Self-Help Revolution*, edited by Frank Riessman and Alan Gartner. New York: Human Sciences Press.

Wilson, Judy. 1995. *How to Work with Self-Help Groups: Guidelines for Professionals*. Hants, England: Arena.

Winicott, D. W. 1958. *Collected Papers*. London: Tavistock.

Withorn, Ann. 1994. Helping ourselves. In *The Sociology of Health and Illness: Critical Perspectives*, edited by Peter Conrad and Rochelle Kern. 4th ed. New York: St. Martin's Press.

Wojtyla, Karol. 1976. The intentional act and the human act: That is, act and experience. In *The Yearbook of Phenomenological Research*, vol. 5, edited by Anna-Teresa Tymieniecka and Analecta Husserliana. Dordrecht: D. Reidel Publishers.

———. 1977. Participation or alienation. In *The Yearbook of Phenomenological Research*, vol. 6, edited by Anna-Teresa Tymieniecka and Analecta Husserliana. Dordrecht: D. Reidel Publishers.

Wollert, R. 1990. Self-help clearinghouses: An overview of an emergent system for promoting mutual aid. In *Working with Self-Help*, edited by Thomas Powell. Silver Spring, Md.: National Association of Social Workers Press.

Wong, Donna, and Cecilia Chan. 1994. Advocacy on self-help for patients with chronic illness: The Hong Kong experience. In *Self-Help and Mutual Aid Groups: International and Multicultural Perspectives*, edited by Francine Lavoie, Thomasina Borkman, and Benjamin Gidron. New York: Haworth Press.

Wuthnow, Robert. 1994. *Sharing the Journey: Support Groups and America's New Quest for Community*. New York: Free Press.

Yalom, Irvin D. 1985. *The Theory and Practice of Group Psychotherapy*. 3rd ed. New York: Basic Books.

Yoshida, Karen K. 1998. Reshaping of self: A pendular reconstruction of self and identity among adults with traumatic spinal cord injury. In *Readings in Medical Sociology*, edited by William C. Cockerham, Michael Glasser, and Linda Heuser. Upper Saddle River, N.J.: Prentice Hall.

Zohar, Asaf, and Thomasina Borkman. 1996. Self-organizing learning organizations: A case study of Alcoholics Anonymous. Paper presented at the 25th annual conference of the Association for Research on Nonprofit Organizations and Voluntary Action. November 9. New York City.

———. 1997. Emergent order and self-organization: A case study of Alcoholics Anonymous. *Nonprofit and Voluntary Sector Quarterly* 26 (4): 527–552.

Zola, Irving Kenneth. 1972. Medicine as an institution of social control. *Sociological Review* 20 (November): 487–504.

———. 1982. *Missing Pieces: A Chronicle of Living with a Disability*. Philadelphia: Temple University Press.

———. 1987. The politicization of the self-help movement. *Social Policy* 18 (Fall): 32–33.

Index

About the Author

Thomasina Jo Borkman received her Ph.D. in sociology from Columbia University in 1969. She began teaching sociology at Catholic University of America in 1969. In 1974 she joined the Department of Sociology and Anthropology, George Mason University in Fairfax, Virginia, where she is now a professor. Her teaching specialties are the sociology of health and illness, small group dynamics, sociology of organizations, human services in society, and deviant behavior.

She has been doing research on self-help groups since 1970, when she began participant observation on a group for people who stutter. She has studied self-help groups of various types continuously since then. As a visiting researcher at the National Institute of Alcohol Abuse and Alcoholism (NIAAA) between 1978 and 1980 she became acquainted with Alcoholics Anonymous and self-help agencies that used AA ideas and organizational principles; she conducted a study of two of these "social model recovery programs," and her monograph on them was published by NIAAA in 1983. She learned firsthand about the experiential knowledge self-helpers gain by participating in a woman's consciousness-raising group in 1972–1973.

She was invited to be on the planning committee for then Surgeon General Everett C. Koop's Workshop on Self-Help and Public Health held in 1978; from this she directed a grant that enabled an advisory group of experts on self-help/mutual aid to convene at the invitation of Surgeon General Koop. She has been an adviser or consultant on self-help groups to various federal agencies, including NIAAA, the National Institutes of Mental Health, and Center for Substance Abuse Treatment. She has also advised or consulted with self-help resource centers or research projects on self-help in Canada, England, North Ireland, and Sweden.

She received a Fulbright Research Fellowship to the Voluntary Action Centre at York University, Toronto, in 1995. Most recently she was awarded an Aspen Nonprofit Institute Research grant to study self-help resource centers in relation to public policy in the United States and Canada. She has written dozens of journal articles on self-help/mutual aid groups. She is especially known for her concept of experiential knowledge, described in a 1976 article in *Social Service Review*. She has edited or co-edited four books or special issues of journals on self-help/mutual aid.